Romona Devi Govender

Suicidal Ideation in HIV-infected persons in South Africa

AF154045

Romona Devi Govender

Suicidal Ideation in HIV-infected persons in South Africa

LAP LAMBERT Academic Publishing

Impressum / Imprint

Bibliografische Information der Deutschen Nationalbibliothek: Die Deutsche Nationalbibliothek verzeichnet diese Publikation in der Deutschen Nationalbibliografie; detaillierte bibliografische Daten sind im Internet über http://dnb.d-nb.de abrufbar.
Alle in diesem Buch genannten Marken und Produktnamen unterliegen warenzeichen-, marken- oder patentrechtlichem Schutz bzw. sind Warenzeichen oder eingetragene Warenzeichen der jeweiligen Inhaber. Die Wiedergabe von Marken, Produktnamen, Gebrauchsnamen, Handelsnamen, Warenbezeichnungen u.s.w. in diesem Werk berechtigt auch ohne besondere Kennzeichnung nicht zu der Annahme, dass solche Namen im Sinne der Warenzeichen- und Markenschutzgesetzgebung als frei zu betrachten wären und daher von jedermann benutzt werden dürften.

Bibliographic information published by the Deutsche Nationalbibliothek: The Deutsche Nationalbibliothek lists this publication in the Deutsche Nationalbibliografie; detailed bibliographic data are available in the Internet at http://dnb.d-nb.de.
Any brand names and product names mentioned in this book are subject to trademark, brand or patent protection and are trademarks or registered trademarks of their respective holders. The use of brand names, product names, common names, trade names, product descriptions etc. even without a particular marking in this work is in no way to be construed to mean that such names may be regarded as unrestricted in respect of trademark and brand protection legislation and could thus be used by anyone.

Coverbild / Cover image: www.ingimage.com

Verlag / Publisher:
LAP LAMBERT Academic Publishing
ist ein Imprint der / is a trademark of
OmniScriptum GmbH & Co. KG
Heinrich-Böcking-Str. 6-8, 66121 Saarbrücken, Deutschland / Germany
Email: info@lap-publishing.com

Herstellung: siehe letzte Seite /
Printed at: see last page
ISBN: 978-3-659-64241-8

Zugl. / Approved by: Durban, University of KwaZulu-Natal, Dissertation, 2013

IDENTIFICATION OF SUICIDAL IDEATION IN HIV-INFECTED PATIENTS: DEVELOPMENT OF A SUICIDE RISK ASSESSMENT TOOL AND A SUICIDE INTERVENTION PLAN FOR HIV- INFECTED PATIENTS FOLLOWING VOLUNTARY COUNSELLING AND TESTING

by

DR. ROMONA DEVI GOVENDER

DEDICATION

I dedicate my PhD to my late husband, Si, who has been my inspiration and emotional support.

ACKNOWLEDGEMENTS

My heartfelt gratitude goes to my late husband, Si, who had started me on my PhD journey. Finishing this manuscript is bitter sweet because he is not here to share my success; but, I have my girls, Ginger and Katy, who took the reins from their dad and encouraged me to finish. Ginger and Katy, you have been my reason to continue and to reach my dream.

I owe my growth and development in research capacity to my supervisor, Professor Lourens Schlebusch. I will forever be grateful to Mrs Tonya Esterhuizen, my biostatistician, without whom the data presented herein may have had no relevance. Together, we have had five publications that have arisen from this thesis.

To my family and friends, many thanks for your support and encouragement.

I wish to extend a huge thank-you to my research participants, without whom this research would not have been possible. I do hope that their participation will make a difference to suicide prevention. My research assistant, Nellie Duma, has been an invaluable link in my PhD, and Mrs P Pillay is acknowledged for her administrative support.

Finally, I gratefully acknowledge financial support from the Columbia University-South African Fogarty AIDS International Training and Research Programme (AITRP) funded by the Fogarty International Center, National Institutes of Health (grant D43TW00231), and a Doctoral Research Grant Award (2010) funded by the University of KwaZulu-Natal.

--
RDG

TABLE OF CONTENTS

ABSTRACT

Background. Globally, suicide and HIV/AIDS remain two of the greatest healthcare issues, particularly in low- and middle-income countries where approximately 85% of suicides occur. Every year, more than 800,000 people die from suicide; this roughly corresponds to one death every 40 seconds, and the World Health Organization (WHO) estimates that by 2020 the rate of death will increase to one every 20 seconds. HIV/AIDS patients in South Africa have a higher suicide risk than the general population and may an increased frequency and severity of suicidal ideation depending on the different intervals in the continuum of HIV disease progression. Several studies have observed a relationship between the increase in suicide and HIV in South Africa, but due to the paucity of empirical data, this relationship remains inconclusive. Suicide in HIV-infected persons is multifactorial. Risk factors include: a history of attempted suicide; fears of social isolation; feelings of hopelessness; fear of losing control of life; elevated levels of depression; denial; and poor coping strategies. Despite the introduction of antiretroviral therapy (ART), the suicide rate remains more than three times higher among HIV-infected persons than in the general population. Although international findings on the correlation between suicide and HIV/AIDS are diverse, results show compelling evidence to screen for suicide risk and intervene as early as possible.

Objectives. The main objectives of this research were: (*i*) to determine the prevalence of suicidal ideation in HIV-positive persons following voluntary HIV counselling and testing (VCT); (*ii*) **to** develop and validate a suicide risk screening scale (SRSS) for use in HIV-infected persons post HIV diagnosis; (*iii*) to implement and evaluate a brief suicide preventive intervention (BSPI) for use in the period immediately following HIV diagnosis.

Methods. A quantitative methodology was used with a cross-sectional, correlational and regression analysis in the prevalence study. Participants completed a sociodemographic questionnaire, Beck's Hopeless Scale and Beck's Depression Inventory. Drawing 14 items from two established screening tests, the SRSS was developed and assessed. Validity, internal consistency and receiver-operating curves were used to determine the sensitivity and specificity of the tool. Following confirmation that recently diagnosed HIV-positive persons were at risk for suicidal behaviour, a BSPI was implemented and its efficacy evaluated with the validated SRSS. Statistical analysis included generalised linear modeling, and Pearson's and McNemar's chi-square analyses.

Results. There was an increase in suicidal ideation over a six-week period following a positive HIV diagnosis, from 17.1% to 24.1%. Suicidal ideation was significantly associated with seropositivity, age and gender, with the majority of affected patients falling in the younger age category. Young males had an 1.8 times higher risk for suicidal ideation than females. Lower education and traditional beliefs were also significantly associated with an HIV-positive status upon testing. The SRSS was implemented and, despite certain limitations, was considered to be a valuable screening tool for suicidal ideation at VCT clinics. The BSPI was associated with a clinically significant decrease in the rate of suicidal ideation over time, providing preliminary evidence on its efficacy.

Conclusion. Significant correlations exist between hopelessness, depression and suicidal ideation; these serve as important markers that should alert healthcare professionals to underlying suicide risks in HIV-positive patients. Screening for suicide risk and possible suicidal behaviour should form a routine aspect of comprehensive patient care at VCT clinics to assist with effective prevention and treatment. Healthcare workers at VCT clinics should be trained in suicide prevention interventions and the importance of educating vulnerable HIV-positive patients on suicide-prevention strategies. Further longitudinal studies are recommended to enable researchers to observe and differentiate between the variables that may be more prevalent at different stages of HIV, as well as the impact of ART on suicidal behaviour.

KEYWORDS

Suicidal ideation; HIV; risk factors; protective factors; suicide; depression; hopelessness; suicide risk assessment; suicide prevention; suicide intervention.

LIST OF ABBREVIATIONS

ARVs   antiretrovirals
ART   antiretroviral therapy
AUC   area under the curve
BDI   Beck's Depression Inventory
BHS   Beck's Hopelessness Scale
BSPI   brief suicide preventive intervention
CI   confidence interval
HIV   human immunodeficiency virus
NIMSS   National Injury Mortality Surveillance System
PLWHA   people living with HIV/AIDS
PTSD   post-traumatic stress disorder
ROC   receiver operating characteristic
RR   risk ratio
SD   standard deviation
SPTC   standard post-test counselling
SRSS   suicide risk screening scale
STDs   sexually transmitted diseases
TB   tuberculosis
WHO   World Health Organization
VCT   voluntary HIV counselling and testing

LIST OF PUBLICATIONS

Govender RD, Schlebusch L. Hopelessness, depression and suicidal ideation in HIV-positive persons. *South African Journal of Psychiatry* 2012; 18(1): 16-21.

Govender RD, Schlebusch L. Suicidal ideation in seropositive patients seen at a south african HIV voluntary counselling and testing clinic. *African Journal of Psychiatry* 2012; 15: 94-98.

Schlebusch L, Govender RD. Age, gender and suicidal ideation following voluntary HIV counselling and testing. *International Journal of Environmental Research and Public Health* 2012; 9: 521-530.

Govender RD, Schlebusch L. A suicide risk screening scale for HIV-infected persons in the immediate post-diagnosis period. *Southern African Journal of HIV Medicine* 2013; 14(2): 58-63.

Govender RD, Schlebusch L, Esterhuizen T. Brief suicide preventive intervention in newly diagnosed HIV-positive persons. *African Journal of Psychiatry* 2014;17: 543-547

CONTRIBUTIONS
The researcher designed and developed all phases of the research protocols, performed all literature searches, secured funding, sought and obtained ethical permissions, trained all staff involved in implementation of the research protocols, performed data capturing, made major contributions to the aforementioned journal publications and prepared the final manuscripts for publication. This is confirmed and supported in the supervisor's report.

CHAPTER 1
ORIENTATION AND PROBLEM STATEMENT

This chapter provides an overview of, and rationale for the study.

1.1 BACKGROUND

Suicide and HIV/AIDS alone are a burden; together, they represent a global crisis and a public health catastrophe. Research has shown that HIV/AIDS patients are at high risk for suicide (Schlebusch and Vawda, 2010). According to the World Health Organization (WHO), over one million people die each year as a consequence of suicide, and in the past 45 years global suicide rates have increased by 60% (WHO, 2008). The latest trends of the global HIV/AIDS epidemic show that the number of people living with HIV rose from around 8 million in 1990 to 34 million by the end of 2010, with sub-Saharan Africa carrying the greatest burden of the epidemic (68% of all HIV-positive people) (AVERT, 2011).

The 2006 National HIV and Syphilis Prevalence Survey in South Africa estimated that the overall HIV prevalence in South Africa was 29.1%, with KwaZulu-Natal Province bearing the highest individual prevalence of 39.1% (NDoH, 2007). Durban, a city in KwaZulu-Natal, is known to be the very hub of the epidemic, with one of the highest HIV-seropositive prevalence rates globally. Some of the South African studies on suicide and HIV have been conducted in this city (UNAIDS, 2006; Schlebusch and Vawda 2010); however, no prior study has focused specifically on the relationship between HIV/AIDS and suicidal ideation in this region. Nevertheless, statistics based on reported attempted suicide have revealed a 25.4% prevalence of suicidal ideation among the general population (UNAIDS, 2006), and a 27% and 73% suicide risk among male and female HIV-positive patients, respectively (Schlebusch and Vawda, 2010).

The pattern of suicidal behaviour may differ throughout the progression of HIV infection up to the development of AIDS. Early international studies have described higher rates of suicidal ideation in HIV-positive individuals (Carrico, *el al.*, 2007) whereas some asymptomatic HIV-infected persons had higher rates of suicidal ideation than persons with AIDS (Kelly, *et al.*, 1998) while some reported suicidal ideation in patients within the first week of testing for HIV (Perry, *el al.*, 1990; Cooperman and Simoni, 2005). Local data reported high levels of suicidal ideation associated with pregnancy, age as well as current and previous depression (Rochat, 2013). There is limited evidence about the prevalence of suicide risk immediately

~ 12 ~

following a positive HIV diagnosis. Consequently, the purpose of this research was to assess suicide risk following voluntary HIV counselling and testing (VCT). VCT offers patients the knowledge to comprehend their HIV status and, depending on the results of testing, affords the ability to access treatment and ultimately presents an opportunity for patients to alter risk behaviour.

1.2 CONCEPT CLARIFICATION

In promoting a clear comprehension of this study in its totality, certain core terms must be clarified:

Suicidal ideation is defined as having the intent to commit suicide, wanting to take one's own life or thinking about suicide without actually making plans to commit suicide (Schlebusch, 2005).

Hopelessness is defined as a feeling that nothing, neither internal resource nor external force, can extricate one from a bleak and unresponsive environment or an experience of despair or extreme pessimism about the future (Beck *et al.*, 1974; Abramson *et al.*, 1990).

Major depressive episode: The essential feature of a major depressive episode is a period of at least 2 weeks during which there is either a depressed mood or loss of interest or pleasure in all activities. The mood in a major depressive episode is often described by the person as 'depressed', 'sad', 'hopeless', 'discouraged' or 'down in the dumps'. The criteria for a major depressive episode include five or more of the symptoms (as listed below) present during the same two-week period and represent a change from previous functioning. The criteria are based on the *Diagnostic and Statistical Manual of Mental Disorders (Fourth Edition, Text Revision)* (DSM-IV-TR) (APA, 2000):

- A depressed mood most of the day, nearly every day, as indicated by either a subjective report or observation made by others;
- A markedly diminished interest or pleasure in all, or almost all activities most of the day, nearly every day;
- Significant weight loss when not dieting, or weight gain, or decrease or increase in appetite nearly every day;
- Insomnia or hypersomnia nearly every day;
- Psychomotor agitation or retardation nearly every day;
- Fatigue or loss of energy nearly every day;
- Feelings of worthlessness or excessive or inappropriate guilt;

- Diminished ability to think or concentrate, or indecisiveness, nearly every day;
- Recurrent thoughts of death, recurrent suicidal ideation without a specific plan, or a suicide attempt or a specific plan for committing suicide.

Following on the WHO/EURO Multicentre Study on Suicidal Behaviour, much debate in the field of suicidology arose regarding the terminology and definitions of suicidal behaviour (De Leo D, *et al.*, 2006) and the inter-relation of suicidal thought, plans and attempts in culturally different societies (Bertolote JM, 2005).

Suicidal behaviour is complex and includes fatal and non-fatal suicidal behaviour, with and without injuries (De Leo D, *et al.*, 2006)

Non-fatal suicidal behaviour, with or without injuries, is defined as "a nonhabitual act with nonfatal outcome that the individual, expecting to, or taking the risk to die or to inflict bodily harm, initiated and carried out with the purpose of bringing about wanted changes" (De Leo D, *et al.*, 2006) For the purpose of this study, includes the following **suicidal ideation** is defined as having the intent to commit suicide, wanting to take one's own life or thinking about suicide without actually making plans to commit suicide (Schlebusch, 2005).

Fatal suicide is often also referred to as **completed suicide** when the individual's intent is to end to his/her own life and he/she ultimately succeeds (Schlebusch, 2005).

1.3 THE HIV EPIDEMIC

HIV/AIDS is the scourge of the 21st century globally. Since the beginning of the HIV epidemic, almost 70 million people have been infected with the virus and about 35 million people have died of AIDS-related causes. Although the burden of the epidemic continues to vary considerably between countries and regions, sub-Saharan Africa remains the most severely affected, with nearly 1 in every 20 adults (4.9%) living with HIV, accounting for 69% of the people living with HIV/AIDS (PLWHA) worldwide. The current estimated total HIV prevalence for South Africa is 5.258 million, with KwaZulu-Natal bearing the highest proportion of this load (15%) (ASSA, 2012).

The overall growth of the HIV epidemic has stabilised in recent years. The annual number of new infections has steadily declined, and due to the significant increase in people receiving antiretroviral therapy (ART), the number of AIDS-related deaths has also diminished (AVERT, 2011). Despite the introduction of ART for

HIV/AIDS patients in South Africa in 2004, HIV is still associated with a very high morbidity and mortality in the country, with 320 000 estimated deaths in 2005 alone (UNAIDS, 2006). The estimated number of people living with HIV in South Africa was 5.6 million at the end of 2009 (UNAIDS, 2012).

1.4 HIV STIGMA AND DISCRIMINIATION

It is well known that PLWHA experience stigma and discrimination on an ongoing basis. At an individual level, stigma undermines a person's identity and capacity to cope with the disease, limits the possibility of disclosure and hinders an eventual alteration in risk behaviour. Closely linked to stigmatisation are discrimination and the disclosure of an individual's HIV status. Stigmatisation and discrimination are inherent within South Africa's history, as depicted by the apartheid system with respect to race. The attachment of discrimination to illness also has a long history, affecting people with mental illness and physical disorders such as cancer, tuberculosis (TB), sexually transmitted diseases (STDs) and leprosy (Sontag, 1988). So, the assumption that discrimination and stigma arise easily within the South African society may not be too unrealistic.

South Africa has reported a large number of incidents of stigma. Blame is often assigned to black people or to women, and some men apportion blame onto women for infecting them with, or spreading HIV (Leclerc-Madlala, 2002). In couples, this can lead to violence against women or their exclusion from the household (Leclerc-Madlala, 2002). The murder of Mpho Mtloung and her mother by her husband, who then also committed suicide, is testimony of such violence towards self and others (TAC, 2002). This type of reaction inevitably has the unfavourable outcome of rendering the epidemic 'invisible' and forcing people who have contracted HIV, or those who are associated with it 'to go into hiding'. The slogan 'Break the Silence', adopted at the International AIDS Conference in Durban in July 2000, was a response to the reluctance of individuals who are HIV-positive to test for HIV and to disclose their HIV status (Morrell, 2001). The manner in which each person experiences and copes with the illness is reflected in their decision of whether or not to disclose their sero-status, and their right to personal privacy and dignity.

1.5 SUICIDE: EPIDEMIOLOGY AND PREVALENCE

Suicidology was first introduced by Shneidman into the English scientific literature in 1964 (Hatton and Valente, 1989). Despite all the research into the subject over the years, suicidology is still surrounded by an aura of mystery. The quest to understand suicide traverses from the sociological theories of Durkheim to the psychoanalytical theories of Freud.

Suicide is a global phenomenon, with the WHO documenting an increasing trend in terms of prevalence (WHO, 2008). In 1998, suicide was estimated to constitute 1.8% of the total global disease burden, with the present global mortality rate estimated to be 14/100 000 (18/100 000 among males and 11/100 000 among females) (WHO, 2008). An increase of up to 1.53 million suicides per annum is projected for the year 2020 (Bertolote and Fleischmann, 2009). Current suicide statistics are even more worrisome when perceived in real-time; e.g. a 16/100 000 global mortality rate translates into one death every 40 seconds (WHO, 2008).

The suicide statistics for South Africa are even more alarming. There are at least 8 attempts for every fatal suicide (Schlebusch, 2004). When compared with international rates, these statistics were deemed higher than the global average (Schlebusch, 2004). Of further concern, it is believed that the South African statistics for completed suicides are not accurate, and that the reported rates are lower than the actual rates. This may be attributed to an evolving vital statistics database, the taboo and stigma related to suicide and, most likely, the misclassification of deaths by suicide. Statistics on fatal suicides are gleaned from a research-based database, the South African National Injury Mortality Surveillance System (NIMSS) (NIMSS, 2007), and data from the Durban Parasuicide Study (PDS) (Schlebusch, 2004). The general trend is that fatal suicides are on the increase (Schlebusch, 2005), and the latest report from NIMSS showed that deaths by suicide constituted 10.71% of the overall deaths in South Africa (NIMSS, 2007). If Durkheim had been asked to comment, he might have described the South African society as being in a state of deep crisis, both at a societal and individual level, with the extremely high prevalence of HIV/AIDS and increasing prevalence of suicide (Schlebusch, 2005).

Suicidal behaviour in the general population may be attributed to multiple factors (Schlebusch, 2005), including genetic, biological, cultural, psychological and social factors, and all of these may contribute either individually or in an interrelated manner, resulting in a cascade of emotional responses. A number of psychosocial risk factors – *viz.* marital disruption, unemployment, lower socioeconomic status, living alone, a recent migration, early parental deprivation, a family history of suicidal behaviour and psychopathology, poor physical health and stressful life events – have been reported to be associated significantly with the risk of suicide (Robertson et al., 2006). These risk factors have been researched extensively internationally and locally (Schlebusch, 2004, 2005; Schlebusch and Vawda, 2010; NIMSS, 2007).

Recent statistics for South Africa have indicated that there has been a shift in the prevalence of suicide, from an act more commonly committed by the elderly, to something that the younger generation is more likely to commit (Schlebusch, 2005). The grounds for suicidal behaviour stem from a constellation of complex components; how these interact or trigger a suicidal outcome may vary from one individual to another (Schlebusch, 2006). The likelihood of suicide or suicidal behaviour has been shown to increase with a higher number of risk factors (Schlebusch, 2006). The greatest risk for suicidal behaviour occurs when risk factors co-exist in individuals and families; yet, the paradox is that individuals may have one or more risk factors but may not be suicidal. Compounding all the complexities of suicide related to genetic, biomedical and psychosocial contributors, South Africa has the added trauma associated with a post-apartheid society, the political transformation that commenced in 1994, and the HIV/AIDS pandemic.

1.6 SUICIDAL IDEATION AND HIV

Are people living with HIV at greater risk for suicide? In South Africa, and on the African continent in general, HIV-related suicide is poorly researched and the relevant statistics are not accurate. In the few studies conducted in South Africa, 16% of the general in-patient admissions for suicidal behaviour were HIV/AIDS-related (Schlebusch, 2006) and the calculated descriptive attempted suicide rate (based on the estimated national suicidal behaviour prevalence rates) was 67.2/100 000 (Schlebusch and Vawda, 2010). As early as 1995, a study in South Africa showed that 17% of youth had attempted suicide because of an AIDS phobia (Mhlongo and Peltzer, 1999).

When patients are first diagnosed with HIV, many react with disbelief and anxiety, and express fear for what lies ahead. Evidence suggests that as many as one half of HIV-positive individuals attempt suicide within three months of notification of their positive status, and about two-thirds do so within the first year (Robertson, 2006; Carrico, 2007; Schlebusch and Vawda, 2010; Kinyanda et al., 2012).

PLWHA may become increasingly suicidal upon a deterioration in their medical condition – e.g. a drop in $CD4^+$ count, an increase in viral load, an opportunistic infection, hospitalisation, pain or the commencement of ART, which may trigger neurocognitive impairment and suicidal thinking (Morrell 2001; Schlebusch and Vawda, 2010; Kinyanda et al., 2012). This is ultimately what laid the foundations for the research described in this dissertation. With the introduction of ART, there may also be an improvement in health which may translate into a decrease in suicide risk, as documented in some international studies; however, this remains to be tested in South Africa (ASSA, 2012).

HIV infection, besides having horrendous and debilitating physical and biological effects, also has a multitude of associated psychosocial impacts (Carrico et al., 2007), which are just as important in determining the risk of suicidal behaviour in HIV-positive persons (ASSA, 2012). Some of the characteristics for suicidality in HIV/AIDS persons in a study conducted in Uganda included female gender, food insecurity, an increase in negative life events, a high stress score, a negative coping style, a past psychiatric history, psychosocial impairment, a diagnosis of post-traumatic stress disorder (PTSD), generalised anxiety disorder and major depressive disorder (Kinyanda et al., 2012). The psychosocial effects can be seen among individuals, families and the community at large, affecting all strata of society and societal functioning, with the ultimate consequence on HIV prevention and treatment. The critical psychosocial stressors for persons with HIV/AIDS follow the same patterns as the general population, with negative effects generated by taboos, social stigma, decreased support from family and friends, multiple losses of family contracting HIV, social devaluation, and so forth, and these negative effects ultimately enhance suicide risk (Robertson et al., 2006; Carrico et al., 2007; Schlebusch and Vawda, 2010; Kinyanda et al., 2012).

Beck's cognitive model of depression provides a framework for understanding how psychological responses to stressful life events may increase suicide risk (Mhlongo and Peltzer, 1999; Allen, 2003; Beck, 2008). HIV-positive persons commonly experience a variety of chronic, uncontrollable stressors that can contribute cumulatively to the perception that living with this stigmatised illness is hopeless and intolerable. Precipitating events are conceptualised as specific stressful life events that are linked to increased suicide risk (Beck et al., 1993). HIV-positive people are faced with being ostracised by family and friends, hence the incentive to withhold the disclosure of their HIV status. Such individuals are also subjected to stigmatisation and discrimination by the society at large.

A number of other psychosocial risk factors have also been associated significantly with the risk of suicide in HIV-positive people, including marital disruption, unemployment, lower socioeconomic status, living alone, a recent migration, early parental deprivation, family history of suicidal behaviour and psychopathology, poor physical health and stressful life events (Robertson *et al.*, 2006; Schlebusch and Vawda, 2010). The prevalence of depression and anxiety in PLWHA is almost double that of HIV-negative people with the same illnesses (Ciesla and Roberts, 2001). Evidence is growing that this is true of South Africa and other African countries (Ciesla and Roberts, 2001; Olley *et al.*, 2004). Taken together, these psychiatric, biological and social vulnerabilities in HIV-positive persons could accentuate hopelessness and the negative impact of stressful life events, and promote cognitive and behavioural patterns that increase suicide risk.

In summary, the risk factors for suicide are diverse and inter-related, and may be particularly complex in HIV-positive individuals. Despite the diverse correlations between suicide and HIV/AIDS (Olley *et al.*, 2004), there is compelling evidence to justify screening for suicide risk and intervening as early as possible (Olley *et al.*, 2004; Bantjies and van Ommen, 2008; Catalan *et al.*, 2011; Badiee *et al.*, 2012).

1.7 SCREENING FOR SUICIDE RISK

All professionals agree that no one can predict who, when and how people will commit suicide. Attempts to predict suicide produce many false-positive and -negative results. Suicide risk assessment includes individual, clinical, interpersonal, situational and demographic factors that increase or decrease suicide risk. There are a variety of suicide risk assessment methods available to the clinician. Suicide assessment forms, structured and semi-structured suicide scales, questionnaires and checklists may complement, but should not substitute the clinician's assessment (Bantjies and van Ommen, 2008). It has been shown that screening for suicide, even among high-risk populations, ultimately does translate into preventing suicides (Hoven *et al.*, 2009).

1.8 SUICIDE PREVENTION AND INTERVENTION

Suicide prevention is defined as any self-injury-prevention or health-promotion strategy that is generally or specifically aimed at reducing the incidence and prevalence of suicidal behaviours (Rehse and Pukrop, 2003). Suicide intervention includes: early recognition and assessment of risk; immediate response; resource referrals; and follow-up management and treatment of at-risk individuals (Rehse and Pukrop, 2003). A complete and comprehensive preventive model is the universal/selective/indicated (USI) model, which targets the general population, vulnerable populations and persons at high risk for suicide. Universal preventive interventions are directed towards entire populations; selective interventions are directed towards individuals who are at greater risk for suicidal behaviour; and indicated preventions target individuals who have already begun to display self-destructive behaviour (Nordentoft, 2011).

1.9 THEORETICAL FRAMEWORK

The theoretical framework underpinning this research is based on Beck's cognitive model of depression (Allen, 2003; Beck, 2008). This framework describes how hopelessness in general, hopelessness about the future and a poor sense of one's own coping skills may act as mediators for suicidal behaviour in HIV-positive persons. This information-processing model states that systematic negativity which pervades cognitive processes forces a person to view events in a specific way – *viz.* the 'cognitive triad' – which activates symptoms of depression (Allen, 2003). Depression-prone patients develop a negative view of themselves. They see themselves as being worthless, unlovable and deficient; they have a negative view of their environment, seeing it as overwhelming, filled with obstacles and failure; and they have a negative view of their future, seeing it as hopeless and believing that no effort will change their lives. This negative way of thinking eventually leads to hopelessness and depression, and ultimately, to suicidal behaviour (Beck *et al.*, 1993).

The supposition is that there is a need to understand the relationship between hopelessness, depression and suicidal behaviour. This relationship has been studied extensively. Hopelessness has been shown to correlate positively with the severity of depression, the number of previous suicide attempts, current suicidal ideation and suicidal intent. In alignment with the present research, this process is illustrated in Fig. 1, overleaf.

Consequently, it is evident that hopelessness is the primary mediator that links depression and suicidal behaviour. One of the best predictors of subsequent suicide is hopelessness, as measured by Beck's Hoplessness Scale (BHS) and the suicide item in Beck's Depression Inventory (BDI) (Beck *et al.*, 1990). Although the correlation between hopelessness, depression and suicide has been well documented, psychosocial characteristics that could ultimately predict suicide in HIV-positive patients need to be interrogated further.

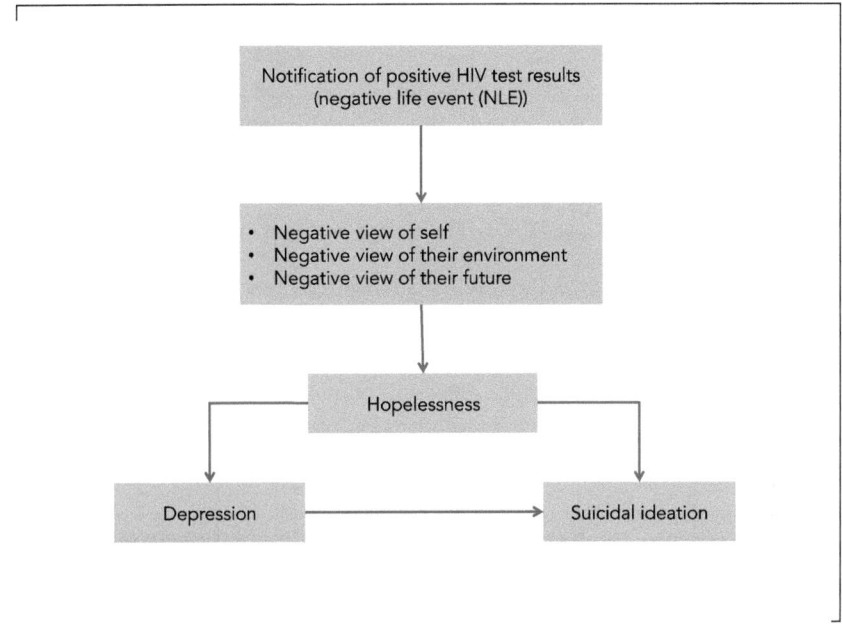

diagnosis, hopelessness, depression and the potential for suicidal ideation.

1.10 RATIONALE FOR THE RESEARCH

The researcher's journey towards a PhD started with a Columbia University-South African Fogarty AIDS International Training and Research Programme scholarship award. This scholarship thrust the researcher into the realms of HIV, and with a background in Family Medicine it was natural to be drawn into researching the impact of psychosocial factors in HIV-positive persons; of course notwithstanding the researcher was practising in a province that has the highest HIV prevalence and is the epicentre of the HIV epidemic in South Africa. It is well documented that HIV-positive persons are suicidal at various stages of HIV disease progression, but little is known about the impact of being told, 'You are HIV-positive' and the cascade of emotions that this statement triggers. To begin to understand the emotional impact, the research done by Beck on the Cognitive Triad of Depression, as well as the related assessment tools developed to assess hopelessness and depression, were considered to be fascinating, especially when Beck was able ultimately to predict suicide using the hopelessness score.

The relationship between HIV/AIDS and suicide has, in the past, been under-researched in developing countries such as South Africa. The risk of suicidal ideation in HIV-positive persons is increasing, as correlated with the HIV pandemic and an increased prevalence of suicide attempts and completed suicides in South Africa (Meel and Leenaars, 2005). Despite the difficulties in determining the prevalence of suicide in HIV-positive patients in South Africa, there has been a parallel increase in suicide and HIV/AIDS mortality (Meel and Leenaars, 2005).

There is a need to understand the risk for suicide and suicidal ideation following notification of a positive HIV-test result, especially immediately post HIV counselling and testing. Therefore, the broad objective of this study was to add to the body of knowledge on suicidal ideation following notification of a positive HIV-test result, and to determine the sociodemographic and psychosocial indicators that may trigger HIV-positive persons to become suicidal.

The theoretical framework underpinning this research assessed the impact of a negative life event, i.e. receiving a positive HIV-test result, and the resultant cascade of emotions, including hopelessness and depression. Hopelessness and depression and their relationship to suicidal behaviour have been studied at length in the general population. In this research, the objective was to test if the same relationship exists in recently diagnosed HIV-positive persons. Beck's Hopelessness Scale (BHS) (Beck, 1974) and Beck's Depression Inventory (BDI) (Beck *et al.*, 1996) were chosen as the screening instruments, as these were internationally validated across different ethnic and cultural societies.

The use of the BHS and BDI allowed for the determination of the rates of hopelessness and depression in the cohort studied, at baseline, 72 hours and 6 weeks after obtaining the HIV-test results. In international research, hopelessness has shown to exhibit a significant correlation with suicide; based on this, the prevalence for suicidal ideation was determined. Although it is known that depression is also associated with suicidal behaviour, this research tested the hypothesis that depression may be used to predict suicidal ideation in recently diagnosed HIV-positive persons.

For practical application of the research findings, the study further sought to develop a suicide risk screening scale (SRSS) – a shortened version of the BHS and BDI – and test its validity and internal consistency in screening recently diagnosed HIV-positive persons for suicidal ideation. The rationale was to develop a self-administered, quick and simple screening scale to identify HIV-positive patients at high risk for suicidal ideation which may be used in under-resourced settings without the need for additional trained staff. This allowed the identification of at-risk individuals requiring intervention and further saw the development of a brief suicide preventive intervention (BSPI) to be used following a positive HIV diagnosis. The BSPI, in turn, was assessed using the validated SRSS at baseline, 72 hours and 6 weeks after a positive HIV diagnosis. The study also evaluated which sociodemographic factors were risk factors and which were protective factors in terms of suicidal ideation.

In summary, five key questions underpinned the research:

1. What is the relationship between hopelessness, depression and suicidal ideation, and can depression be used to predict suicidal ideation?
2. What is the prevalence of suicidal ideation in HIV-positive persons following VCT?
3. What is the relationship between sociodemographic factors and suicidal ideation following VCT?
4. Can a brief SRSS be used to screen recently diagnosed HIV-positive persons for suicidality in order to assist with treatment and suicide prevention?
5. What is the effect of a brief psychosocial intervention on suicide risk following a positive HIV test result?

1.11 RESEARCH FOCUS

The overarching aim of this study was to measure the effectiveness of an SRSS among HIV-positive persons in order to implement a BSPI post HIV diagnosis to reduce suicidal ideation in HIV-positive persons following VCT.

The specific goals of this study were to:

- Describe the relationship between sociodemographic factors and suicidal ideation following VCT;
- Determine the prevalence of suicidal ideation at two time-points following VCT;
- Determine whether depression can be used to predict suicidal ideation;
- Develop an SRSS and test its validity, reliability and internal consistency in assessing suicide risk in HIV-positive persons;
- Implement a BSPI plan post HIV diagnosis for HIV-positive persons.

1.12 METHODOLOGY

The methodology is presented independently for the three phases in **Chapters Two**, **Three** and **Four**.

1.12.1 ETHICAL CONSIDERATIONS

Ethical approval for all three phases of the research described herein was obtained from the University of KwaZulu-Natal (UKZN) Biomedical Research and Ethics Committee, the UKZN Postgraduate Committee and the Department of Health.

The study participants were advised of the study either in English or isiZulu as requested; for those that could not read or write, the research assistant provided the necessary support. All research participants' rights (including that to confidentiality) were maintained and only complete voluntary participation was respected. The participants were compensated for their travelling expenses.

In terms of data management and storage, all electronic databases were password-protected and the raw data were kept in a lockable cabinet, to which only the researcher had access.

If the interviewer suspected that a participant was at high risk for suicide, then the relevant referral for help was made for more intensive treatment.

1.13 DELINEATION OF THIS STUDY

Chapter 1 includes an introduction to the research and outlines the rationale for the broader study.

Chapter 2 presents research exploring the relationship between hopelessness, depression and suicidal ideation in HIV-positive persons.

Chapter 3 presents the development of an SRSS via modification of the existing BHS and BDI, and describes the testing of the validity and reliability thereof.

Chapter 4 summarises the development and implementation of a BSPI for inclusion in the standard post-test counselling (SPTC) of HIV-positive persons, and assesses the outcomes of the BSPI using the validated SRSS at baseline, within 72 hours and at 6 weeks.

Chapter 5 summarises the key findings of the broader study and the practical applications thereof, discusses the study limitations, and provides recommendations for future work.

1.14 CONCLUDING REMARKS

An increasing trend of suicide and suicidal behaviour is forecast for the coming years. Society needs to awaken from the 'ostrich head' phenomenon in this regard and take charge of this growing epidemic to decrease suicide prevalence. The sociodemographic factors associated with suicide are a cause for great concern, with younger people being at higher risk, and males classically exhibiting a higher rate for completed suicides. South Africa is not insulated from these statistics; rather, the country suffers rates that are higher than the global average. Furthermore, South Africa has the added impediment of the HIV pandemic. Some statistics are available on the prevalence of suicide in HIV-positive persons, but these are not adequate to estimate the burden of suicide in this national cohort of patients.

Accompanying the burden of a positive HIV diagnosis is a battery of psychosocial issues. The impact of these on suicide counselling needs to be comprehended in order for healthcare professionals to implement effective strategies for management and prevention programmes. HIV-positive persons need to be assessed for suicidal ideation and the underlying psychosocial issues must be addressed in an intervention plan in order to provide effective coping and risk-management skills that could ultimately reduce suicidal

CHAPTER 2

PHASE ONE: PREVALENCE OF SUICIDAL IDEATION IN HIV-POSITIVE PERSONS FOLLOWING VOLUNTARY COUNSELLING AND TESTING

2.1 INTRODUCTION

The objectives of **Phase One** were: (*i*) to determine the prevalence and incidence ratio of suicidal ideation at two time-points following VCT; and (*ii*) to determine the association between depression, hopelessness and suicidal ideation.

Three peer-reviewed scholarly publications arose from Phase One:

- **Article One** was based on the relationship between hopelessness, depression and suicidal ideation following VCT, and therefore the choice of BHS and BDI as assessment tools.
- **Article Two** followed naturally, looking at suicidal ideation and sociodemographic factors.
- **Article Three** described age and gender as risk factors for suicidal ideation, since current research showed a shift away from the elderly being at higher risk for suicidal behaviour, instead to younger persons being at higher risk. Females are known to be greater risk for attempted suicide, and the objective was to determine whether this *status quo* held true for HIV-infected females.

2.2 METHODOLOGY
2.2.1 STUDY DESIGN

Phase One was prospective and observational.

2.2.2 STUDY AREA AND POPULATION

The study sample consisted of adult volunteer patients (N=200) attending the voluntary HIV counselling and testing (VCT) clinic at a university-affiliated, general state hospital in Durban, KwaZulu-Natal, South Africa, over a three-month period. The study was approved by the Biomedical Research Ethics Committee of the University of KwaZulu-Natal and permission was granted by the relevant health institution. The recruited patients signed voluntarily informed consent to participate in the study. Administered questionnaires were completed in the language preferred by each participant preferred (either English or isiZulu).

2.2.3 INSTRUMENTS

2.2.3.1 A BRIEF SOCIODEMOGRAPHIC INVENTORY (ANNEXURE 1)

2.2.3.2 BECK'S HOPELESSNESS SCALE (BHS) (ANNEXURE 2)

BHS is one of the most widely used measures of hopelessness, and addresses three major aspects thereof: feelings about the future; loss of motivation; and expectations. The BHS questionnaire is then scored according to the answers given. The BHS is a 20-item true-false instrument that assesses the degree to which a person holds negative expectations about the future. Nine of the items are keyed false and 11 true. The items are summed to obtain a total hopelessness score, ranging from 0 to 20. The scale has excellent internal consistency and test-retest reliability. The concurrent validity is well established across a wide variety of samples and the scale has frequently been used in treatment-outcome studies. Several studies have supported the predictive validity of BHS for suicide attempts and completed suicide. Psychological well-being is assessed using the following scoring scale: $0 - 3$ (none or minimal); $4 - 8$ (mild); $9 - 14$ (moderate and may not be in immediate danger but requires frequent regular monitoring. Is the life situation stable?); and 15 (severe; definite suicidal risk).

Research consistently supports a positive relationship between the BHS score and measures of depression, suicidal intent and suicidal ideation. Beck found, in a cohort of 1 958 outpatients, that hopelessness – measured according to BHS – was also significantly related to eventual suicide. Thus, BHS may be used as an indicator of suicide potential (Beck et al., 1974, 1990, 1993).

2.2.3.3 BECK'S DEPRESSION INVENTORY (BDI) (ANNEXURE 3)

The BDI consists of 21 items, each consisting of 4 statements that reflect gradations in the intensity of a particular depressive symptom. The respondent chooses the statement that best describes how the respondent feels at the time of responding. The questionnaire is composed of items relating to symptoms of depression, such as hopelessness and irritability; cognition, such as guilt and feeling of being punished; as well as physical symptoms, such as weight loss, fatigue and lack of interest in sex. The first two-thirds of the questions score emotional symptoms and the remaining third physical symptoms. The individual statements are scored from 0 to 3 and the sum total ranges from 0 to 63; $0 - 9$ (not depressed); $10 - 15$ (mildly depressed); $16 - 24$ (moderately depressed); and ≥ 25 (severely depressed).

2.2.4 DATA COLLECTION

A sociodemographic questionnaire was completed following VCT. BHS and BDI were completed within 72 hours and again within 6 weeks to determine the impact of a positive HIV-test result on suicidal ideation.

2.2.5 DATA ANALYSIS

The data were stratified according to age, gender, educational status, professional status, marital status, religion/traditional beliefs and race/ethnicity. The prevalence of suicidal ideation and the suicidal incident ratio were determined. Participants were also assessed for hopelessness and depression at two time intervals.

2.2.6 STATISTICAL ANALYSIS

SPSS software (version 15.0; SPSS Inc, Chicago, Illinois, USA) was used for data analysis. Pearson's chi-squared test, t-tests and a binary logistic regression analysis of the sociodemographic variables were conducted. The latter used a backward stepwise method with entry and exit probabilities set at 0.05 and 0.1 based on likelihood ratio tests. The sociodemographic variables were entered into the model at step one. After five steps, the final model was reported with odds ratios (ORs) and 95% confidence intervals (CIs).

2.3 ARTICLE ONE

Key question: What is the relationship between hopelessness, depression and suicidal ideation, and can depression be used to predict suicidal ideation?

CITATION:

GOVENDER RD, SCHLEBUSCH L. HOPELESSNESS, DEPRESSION AND SUICIDAL IDEATION IN HIV-POSITIVE PERSONS. *SOUTH AFRICAN JOURNAL OF PSYCHIATRY* 2012; 18(1): 16-21.

ABSTRACT:

Background. HIV/AIDS and suicidal behaviour are major public health concerns.

Objective. The aim of this study was to examine the relationship between hopelessness, depression and suicidal ideation in HIV-infected persons.

Methods. The sample consisted of all adult volunteers attending a VCT clinic at a university-affiliated state hospital. Suicidal ideation and depression were measured using BHS and BDI, respectively, at two intervals, *viz.* 72 hours and 6 weeks after HIV diagnosis.

Results. Of the 156 patients who tested positive for HIV, 32 (20.5%) had a hopelessness score of 9 or above on BHS and 130 patients (82.8%) were depressed according to BDI at 72 hours after diagnosis. Of the 109 patients assessed 6 weeks after diagnosis, 32 (28.8%) had a hopelessness score >9 on BHS and 86 (78.2%) were depressed according to BDI. A moderately positive correlation at both time periods was found between hopelessness and depression. A receiver operating characteristic (ROC) analysis showed optimal sensitivity, indicating that the HIV-positive depressed patients were at risk for suicidal behaviour.

Conclusion. The significant correlations between hopelessness, depression and suicidal ideation are important markers that should alert healthcare professionals to underlying suicide risks in HIV-positive patients. Early recognition of this and suicide prevention strategies should be incorporated into the treatment offered at VCT clinics.

2.4 ARTICLE TWO

Key question: What is the prevalence of suicidal ideation in HIV-positive persons following VCT?

CITATION:

GOVENDER RD, SCHLEBUSCH L. SUICIDAL IDEATION IN SEROPOSITIVE PATIENTS SEEN AT A SOUTH AFRICAN HIV VOLUNTARY COUNSELLING AND TESTING CLINIC. *AFRICAN JOURNAL OF PSYCHIATRY* 2012; 15: 94-98.

ABSTRACT:

Objective. Suicidal behaviour and HIV/AIDS are significant public health concerns. The aim of this study was to investigate suicidal ideation in patients who were referred to a VCT clinic and who were found to be seropositive. This is in order to improve suicide prevention and intervention strategies among such patients.

Method. The sample studied consisted of volunteer adult patients referred over a three-month period to an HIV clinic based at a university-affiliated general state hospital. Patients completed a questionnaire on sociodemographic data. Suicidal ideation was measured using BHS and BDI, at two time-points (within 72 hours after notification and again at a six-week follow-up). All patients received extensive pre-and post-test counselling.

Results. HIV-test results were available for 189 (99.5%) of the original sample of 190 patients studied, with 157 (83.1%) testing positive. More females tested positive as did unemployed and single/divorced patients. The mean age for HIV-positive patients was 33.49 years (SD ±9.449), and for HIV-negative patients it was 37.94 years (SD ±15.238). Age was a significant factor in that for each year increase in age, the risk of testing HIV-positive decreased by 4.1%. Lower education and traditional beliefs were also significantly associated with testing HIV-positive. At 72 hours suicidal ideation was present in 17.1% (95% CI 12.16 - 23.45), and at 6 weeks in 24.1% (95% CI 17.26 - 32.39) of the seropositive patients. Their average BDI scores were 15.20 and 14.23, respectively, at the two time-points.

Conclusion. Suicidal ideation was present in a significant number of the seropositive cohort studied and increased over a six-week period among these patients. The average BDI scores at both time points imply a clinical depression. The findings also suggest an association between positive HIV-test results and certain sociodemographic variables that can act as indicators for suicidal ideation in HIV-infected persons, although this requires further research. Although the relationship between suicidal ideation and HIV-infection is complex, it is an important consideration when assessing patient suicide vulnerability at VCT clinics and when implementing suicide prevention and management strategies.

2.5 ARTICLE THREE

Key question: What is the relationship between sociodemographic factors and suicidal ideation following VCT?

CITATION:

SCHLEBUSCH L, GOVENDER RD. AGE, GENDER AND SUICIDAL IDEATION FOLLOWING VOLUNTARY HIV COUNSELLING AND TESTING. *INTERNATIONAL JOURNAL OF ENVIRONMENTAL RESEARCH AND PUBLIC HEALTH* 2012; 9: 521-530.

ABSTRACT:

Objective. The aim of this study was to determine the prevalence of suicidal ideation in patients who were tested for HIV-infection and whether, along with their HIV status, age and gender influenced their risk for suicidal ideation.

Methods. The sample consisted of 189 patients who attended a VCT clinic at a general state hospital in Durban, South Africa. Their mean age at baseline was 34.2 years, with an age range of between 16 and 79 years.

Results. Seropositivity, age and gender were significantly associated with suicidal ideation. The majority of these patients were in the younger age group, and young males had a 1.8 times higher risk for suicidal ideation than females. Although risk factors for seropositive-related suicidal ideation can be complex and multi-factorial, this study identified a young age and male gender as important high risk factors in the sample studied.

Conclusion. It is recommended that all, but especially young male HIV-infected patients seen at VCT clinics are screened for suicidal ideation and that early intervention to prevent subsequent suicides or suicidal attempts are included in pre- and post-test HIV counselling.

~ 31 ~

CHAPTER 3

PHASE TWO: DEVELOPMENT AND VALIDATION OF A SUICIDE RISK SCREENING SCALE FOR USE FOLLOWING A POSITIVE HIV DIAGNOSIS

3.1 INTRODUCTION

The objective of **Phase Two** was to develop an SRSS for suicidal ideation in HIV-positive persons following HIV counselling and testing.

This chapter challenged the researcher. The question beckoned: Can a suicide risk scale be developed without 're-inventing the wheel' and make a lasting contribution to society? The challenges experienced can be summarised as follow: are self-reported assessments or structured interviews more effective and reliable at assessing high-risk persons for suicidal behaviour? The literature also showed that a shortened BHS with either a single-item or a 4-item questionnaire was reliable and valid. Yip and Cheung (2006) conducted a cross-sectional study assessing whether a single item ('My future seems dark to me') and a 4-item component of BHS (including positive and negative items describing the perception of the future in terms of success, darkness, lack of opportunity and faith) could summarise most of the information that BHS provides. Results showed that the 4-item component was a useful alternative to BHS. Shortening of the psychometric instrument should be considered so as to reduce the burden on patients and to improve the response rate (Yip and Cheung, 2006). An item analysis of BHS was conducted, looking specifically at item endorsement and item-total correlations. Three abbreviated versions (3-item, 7-item and 13-item) were developed based on certain denoted item-total correlation cut-offs. Reliability and validity of the original 20-item BHS were then compared with that of the newly developed abbreviated versions. All scales were found to be reliable and valid measures of hopelessness. The three abbreviated versions were more strongly correlated with the distress measures than the original version. The 7- and 13-item subscales outperformed the original BHS in the prediction of suicidal ideation (Abbey *et al.*, 2006).

The results for BDI are supportive of its reliability and validity across various cultures. A brief form consisting of 13 items developed for general practitioner use correlated 0.96 with the total on the standard form and the internal consistency ranged from 0.70 to 0.90. Suicidal ideation can be assessed only on item 9 of BDI (Perry *et al.*, 1990); results suggest that patients who score 2 or higher on the BDI suicide item are 6.9 times (95% CI 3.7 - 12.6) more likely to commit suicide than patients who score less than 2.

In a recent study conducted among HIV-positive persons in South Africa, suicidal ideation increased over a six-week period and was present in 24% of the HIV-positive participants following HIV counselling and testing (Govender *et al.*, 2012). These statistics serve as compelling evidence to assess for suicide risk and intervene as early as possible.

3.2 METHODOLOGY

3.2.1 STUDY DESIGN

Phase Two was a validity and reliability study.

3.2.2 STUDY AREA AND STUDY POPULATION

The sample consisted of HIV-positive adults presenting to an academic, district-level hospital in Durban, KwaZulu-Natal, South Africa. One hundred and fifty consenting participants were enrolled for the validity and reliability testing of an SRSS and participants returned three weeks later for a re-test. The study was approved by the Biomedical Research Ethics Committee of the University of KwaZulu-Natal and permission was granted by the relevant health institution.

3.2.3 INSTRUMENTS

Two well-known and extensively used scales were used to assess aspects of suicidal behaviour in various population groups, *viz.* BHS and BDI. Co-morbid conditions have been found to affect the specificity of severity ratings at both the low- and high-end scores (APA, 2000). Several researchers have used items from both of these scales to validate the use of shorter versions in specific populations (APA, 2000; Yip and Cheung, 2006). For the purposes of the present study, 11 items were selected from BHS and 1 item from consists of 3 different responses to construct a short 14-item SRSS for clinical use in an HIV/AIDS VCT setting (Table 1). The 11 BHS items are negatively phrased questions that represent expectations of failure or motivational components (items 2, 9, 11, 16, 17 and 20), and those that reflect future uncertainty or cognitive components (items 4, 7, 12, 14 and 18). The components that this scale measures have been addressed in previous research (APA, 2000; Aish and Wasserman, 2001). Therefore, the rationale in the present study for item selection incorporated several additional considerations. Firstly, it was considered that those patients with extreme pessimism would endorse the negative items selected and thus be more likely to exhibit suicide risk (Aish and Wasserman, 2001; Yip and Cheung, 2006). Secondly, the item size pool is underscored by a theoretical framework that the patients' perceived hopelessness about their situation and their future could be linked to suicide risk. This stems from the premise that hopelessness is an important psychological and cognitive construct that can be used to predict suicidal risk in a clinical setting (Beck *et al.*, 1974). In line with the scoring of BHS, the 14 items of the SRSS were scored: true = 1; false = 0. A cut-off score greater than or equal to 4 was considered to be positive for suicidal ideation.

3.2.4 STATISTICAL ANALYSIS

3.2.4.1 TEST-RETEST RELIABILITY

A Pearson's correlation coefficient (r) of 0.70 and above deemed the test to be reliable. The SRSS was administered to HIV-positive participants at baseline and 3 weeks thereafter – a time interval shown to have an r-value of 0.79 in detecting content validity and reliability. The scores were correlated against each other using Pearson's correlation coefficient. The coefficient was used to determine the reliability of the SRSS; i.e. the closer to 1, the more reliable the scale.

3.2.4.2 INTERNAL CONSISTENCY

Measures of internal consistency are used to evaluate the extent to which different items on a test measure the same characteristics; i.e. they serve as a measure of agreement among the components of an instrument. This assesses the reliability of the test by assessing consistency among the items as represented by high reliability values. However, low reliability values should not be dismissed and may be acceptable in comparing groups. Different desirable reliability values are quoted for various psychological measurements. The internal consistency of the items that measure these two constructs were tested using Cronbach's alpha. An alpha value greater than or equal to 0.7 was considered to indicate that the scale showed good internal consistency.

3.2.4.3 VALIDITY TESTING: SUPRE-MISS

The WHO Multisite Intervention Study on Suicidal Behaviours (SUPRE-MISS) was launched on five continents (including Durban, South Africa on the African continent) to increase knowledge about suicidal behaviours and effective interventions for those individuals from culturally diverse societies attempting suicide. The SUPRE-MISS instruments were pilot tested, translated into different languages and validated for the prediction of suicidal behaviour. Accordingly, the SUPRE-MISS items which were used to test the validity of the SRSS in the present study were:

1. Have you ever seriously thought about committing suicide?
2. Have you ever made a plan for committing suicide?
3. Have you ever attempted suicide?

The SRSS and SUPRE-MISS were administered to HIV-positive participants at baseline. The SUPRE-MISS was used as the standard to classify participants as either positive or negative for suicidal ideation. Similarly, the SRSS was used to classify the same participants using the cut-off points described above. The results of the two tests were cross-tabulated against each other and sensitivity, specificity and positive and negative predictive values were calculated. This was anticipated to show either convergent or discriminant validity and thus construct validity.

a. ARTICLE 4

Key question: Can a brief suicide risk screening scale be used to screen recently diagnosed HIV-positive persons for suicidality in order to assist with treatment and suicide prevention?

CITATION:

GOVENDER RD, SCHLEBUSCH L. A SUICIDE RISK SCREENING SCALE FOR HIV-INFECTED PERSONS IN THE IMMEDIATE POST-DIAGNOSIS PERIOD. *SOUTHERN AFRICAN JOURNAL OF HIV MEDICINE* 2013; 14(2): 58-63.

ABSTRACT:

The risk of suicidality in HIV-positive persons appears to be significant among vulnerable individuals within the context of the HIV pandemic, and may be paralleled with an increased prevalence of suicidal behaviour in South Africa. The aim of this study was to construct a brief SRSS to screen recently diagnosed HIV-positive persons for suicidality in order to assist with treatment and suicide prevention. The sample consisted of a randomly selected cohort of 150 HIV-positive, consenting adults who presented at an HIV/AIDS VCT clinic at an academic district level hospital in Durban, South Africa. The participants were not taking antiretroviral medication. Participants returned three weeks after their initial assessment for a re-assessment. The SRSS utilised selected items from two established relevant tests and this consisted of 12-items. It was compared with an appropriate psychological instrument that measures suicidality. Inter-item characteristics, internal consistency, reliability and validity were determined. The results were statistically significant and showed adequate sensitivity and specificity. The findings suggest that, despite certain limitations, the SRSS can be used as a valuable screening tool for suicidality at VCT clinics as part of a clinical interview for the assessment of suicide risk. It is recommended that suicide risk assessment should form a routine aspect of comprehensive patient care at such clinics, which can assist with effective prevention and treatment of possible suicidal behaviour in HIV-positive persons.

CHAPTER 4

PHASE THREE: EVALUATION OF A BRIEF SUICIDE PREVENTIVE INTERVENTION FOLLOWING HIV DIAGNOSIS

4.1 INTRODUCTION

The objective of **Phase Three** was to evaluate a brief suicide preventive intervention and assess the outcomes thereof.

4.2 METHODOLOGY

4.2.1 STUDY DESIGN

Phase Three comprised a controlled clinical trial with an experimental arm.

4.2.2 STUDY AREA AND STUDY POPULATION

The study was conducted at Wentworth Hospital, a university-affiliated hospital. Patients aged 18 years and older and who were HIV-positive following VCT were included in the study. Persons who were WHO HIV/AIDS stage 3 and 4 were not considered to be eligible for the study.

Once patients (*N*=129) were diagnosed as being HIV-positive following VCT, they were subjected to SPTC. Thereafter, every alternate participant was given one extra hour of a BSPI. The research protocol was approved by the relevant ethics committee and all enrolled participants gave written informed consent.

4.2.3 STANDARD POST-TEST COUNSELLING

All participants were subjected to the SPTC that is provided to all patients who test HIV-positive. The principles of SPTC include:

1. Delivering the result in a private and confidential manner;
2. The need to discuss with the patient the impact of disclosure of the test result;
3. TEST RESULT: POSITIVE;
4. Telling the patient the result and showing him/her the result;
5. Allowing the patient to digest this information;
6. Giving the patient time to explore his/her feelings and fears; understanding that the client may become emotionally 'shocked'; reassuring him/her that he/she will not be abandoned by the clinician; and explaining that coming to terms with the result may take some time;

7. The need to understand that the health services have much to provide in terms of the different modalities of treatment: 'You can remain healthy if you take care of yourself, eat healthy foods, do not smoke, do not drink, do not take drugs and see a doctor as soon as you feel ill. You can also be given HIV medication that will not cure you, but will keep you healthy. The ART will be given once your $CD4^+$ count drops below 200 cells/µl and you join the ART programme at the hospital. The drugs can also make you sick, but you can be treated if you go early to the hospital or doctor.';

8. Expressing the need to understand the different modes of transmission and how the patient could transmit the virus to others; and encouraging safe sex practices, stressing condom use.

9. Explaining the natural history of the progression of the disease and the intervention programmes available to assist in the patient's treatment and how it can prolong his/her health with a change in lifestyle and treatment programmes;

10. The hospital social worker will be a part of the ART programme and will assist with social support and support resources.

4.2.4 BRIEF SUICIDE PREVENTIVE INTERVENTION (BSPI)

Participants in the intervention group were offered a suicide preventive intervention that included addressing the psychosocial issues related to HIV-positivity at the time of presentation. This therapy entails identifying and helping to resolve interpersonal difficulties that cause or exacerbate psychological distress. The BSPI session was one hour in duration and encompassed the following aspects to render it effective and relevant to the target population:

1. Feedback on the research outcomes regarding the percentage of those who are at risk for suicidal ideation following HIV counselling and testing; risk factors and protective factors were encompassed, together with the manner in which patients should deal with risk factors;

2. Empathy: the situation was seen in light of the person's situation while maintaining objectivity and being non-judgemental;

3. Advice: simple advice on how to live positively;

4. Responsibility: it was considered the responsibility of the person to take the onus to change;

5. Self-efficacy: the person's belief in their ability to make meaningful changes was encouraged;

6. Sociodemographic factors: protective factors;

7. Psychosocial factors: stigmatisation, disclosure and gender issues.

During the session, the pattern of questioning and answering was avoided. This pattern, which gives the impression that the counsellor has all of the answers to all of the questions, might have led the patient to play a passive role, counter to the objective of the BSPI. Importantly, the counsellor continually re-enforced positive counselling and made no attempt to apportion blame or to be judgemental towards the patient.

4.2.5 INFORMATION

4.2.5.1 WHAT IS SUICIDAL IDEATION?

Suicidal ideation is defined as having the intent to commit suicide, wanting to take one's own life or thinking about suicide without actually making plans to commit suicide.

4.2.5.2 HOW MANY PEOPLE THINK ABOUT SUICIDE?

In a recent study (detailed in *section 2.3* of *Chapter Two*), we found that 17.1% of patients had suicidal ideation 72 hours after being told that they were HIV-positive, and 6 weeks thereafter, 24.1% of the same patients were still at risk for suicidal ideation (Govender and Schlebusch, 2012).

4.2.5.3 WHAT PUSHES PEOPLE TOWARDS THINKING ABOUT SUICIDE?

This negative view about a life situation may be intolerable, and suicidal ideation may provide a safety valve for feelings of fear and distress; i.e. it is a path that the affected person feels compelled to take, seeing no way out of his/her problems, pain and misery. In this instance, a counsellor may be required to point out to the patient that there are other ways out, and to assist and support the patient to engage with alternate solutions.

4.2.5.4 RISK FACTORS FOR SUICIDAL IDEATION

4.2.5.4.1 DEPRESSION

Depression is characterised by a feeling of sadness for most of the day. While everyone feels depressed, sad and lonely at certain times, these feelings usually pass. If they persist for longer than two weeks, then the individual needs to seek help. Common symptoms of depression include:

- a markedly diminished interest or pleasure in all, or almost all activities for most of the day, nearly every day;
- significant weight loss when not dieting, or weight gain, or a decrease or increase in appetite nearly every day;
- insomnia or hypersomnia nearly every day;
- psychomotor agitation or retardation nearly every day;
- fatigue or loss of energy nearly every day;
- feelings of worthlessness or excessive or inappropriate guilt;
- a diminished ability to think or concentrate, or indecisiveness, nearly every day;
- recurrent thoughts of death, recurrent suicidal ideation without a specific plan, or a suicide attempt or specific plan for committing suicide.

4.2.5.4.2 GENDER

As detailed in *section 2.5* of *Chapter Two*, among a cohort of patients attending a VCT clinic at a general state hospital in Durban, we found that HIV-positive males had a 1.8 times higher risk for suicidal ideation than females. Cautiously, however, this does not mean that females are *not* at risk (Nock MK, *et al*, 2008; Schlebusch and Govender, 2012).

4.2.5.4.3 AGE

Recent statistics have indicated that there has been a shift in the prevalence of suicidal behaviour in South Africa, from previously, more common among the elderly, to recently, more common among the younger generation (Nock MK, *et al*, 2008; Schlebusch and Vawda, 2010). As detailed in *section 2.5* of *Chapter Two*, we found that as the age of HIV-positive subjects increased by one year (age range 16 - 79 years), the risk for suicidal behaviour increased by a factor of 1.03 (Schlebusch and Govender, 2012). Cautiously, although this means that the older an individual is at the time of a positive HIV diagnosis, the higher the likelihood of experiencing trouble in dealing with the diagnosis and the greater the risk for suicidal ideation, even young people may experience difficulty accepting a positive HIV-test result.

4.2.5.4.4 MARITAL STATUS

In the general population, single, divorced and widowed persons are at greater risk for suicidal behaviour (Nock MK, *et al*, 2008; Fukuchi N *et al.*, 2013). Among HIV-positive persons, however, research has not singled out any marital status that confers a higher risk for suicidal ideation.

4.2.5.4.5 OCCUPATION

In the general population, the loss of a job, rather than being unemployed, has a higher risk for suicide (Blakely TA, *et al.*, 2003; Cooperman, *et al.*, 2005). In HIV-positive persons, however, unemployment has been cited as the major contributory factor among 44% of a cohort who reported suicide risk (Schlebusch L, 2006).

4.2.5.4.6 EDUCATION

There is available statistical data or clinical data to suggest that level of education is a major contributory factor to the suicide potential of an individual (Nock MK, *et al*, 2008; Govender and Schlebusch, 2012).

4.2.5.4.7 MIGRATION

Post-1994 migration is still a way of life for 60% of men in South Africa, and is associated with challenges that may render these men at risk for suicidal ideation. This migration is associated with a degree of emotional instability considering a move from a rural to an urban environment, the loneliness associated with being away from their families, fears that their partners may be unfaithful to them, and fears that their children will grow up without a father's guidance (Hosegood and Timaeus, 2006).

4.2.5.4.8 STIGMATISATION

Being HIV-positive is associated with its own social stigma (Skinner and Mfecane, 2004). Promoting individuals to talk openly about HIV/AIDS, prevention and treatment will help to de-stigmatise this illness.

4.2.5.5 FACTORS PROTECTIVE AGAINST SUICIDAL IDEATION
(Mann,*et al.*, 2005; WHO, 2012)

4.2.5.5.1 FAMILY PATTERNS

Good family patterns have been found to be protective against suicidal ideation, including:

- encouraging good relationships and support from family;
- encouraging family therapy, if agreeable by the patient;
- devoted and consistent parenting.

4.2.5.5.2 COGNITIVE STYLE AND PERSONALITY

Cognitive styles and personalities found to be protective against suicidal ideation include:

- confidence in oneself and one's own situation and achievements;
- a sense of personal value;
- seeking help when difficulties arise;
- seeking advice when important choices must be made;
- openness to other people's experiences and solutions;
- openness to learning;
- an ability to communicate.

4.2.5.5.3 CULTURAL AND SOCIODEMOGRAPHIC FACTORS

Cultural and sociodemographic factors that are protective against suicidal ideation include:

- encouraging good social networking, sporting activities, religious activities, etc.
- higher education and employment – especially for women, but the same applies to men – offers some protection, i.e. it gives women economic power and therefore the ability to negotiate with their male counterparts, to plan a family, to have better socioeconomic status and to have improved healthcare;
- the adoption of specific cultural values and traditions;
- good relationships with friends, workmates, neighbours;
- support from relevant people;
- non-substance-using friends;
- social integration, e.g. through work, participation in sport, different clubs and religious activities;
- a sense of purpose with one's life.

4.2.5.5.4 ENVIRONMENTAL FACTORS

Environmental factors protective against suicidal ideation include:

- a good diet;
- good sleeping patterns;
- exposure to sunlight;
- physical exercise;
- a non-drug, non-smoking environment.

4.2.5.6 WHAT SUPPORT IS AVAILABLE?

If the interviewer identified a participant to be at high risk for suicide, then the relevant referral for help was made for more intensive treatment. Available facilities in the study setting included: a resident clinical psychologist at Wenworth Hospital; the option to admit high-risk patients as in-patients; and LifeLine support services.

4.2.6 OUTCOME MEASURES

The SRSS is a 14-item instrument that assesses suicidal ideation by measuring hopelessness and a patient's thoughts about committing suicide. An SRSS score greater than or equal to 4 was considered to be clinically significant for suicidal ideation.

4.2.7 STATISTICAL ANALYSIS

Strata software (version 12) was used for statistical analysis. Generalised linear modelling was used to categorise participants with suicidal ideation (positive ideation was defined as a score of ≥ 4). Pearson's chi-square test was used to determine the statistical significance of differences between the control and intervention groups. McNemar's chi-square test was used for paired binary proportions.

4.3 ARTICLE FIVE

Key question: What is the effect of a brief psychosocial intervention on suicide risk following a positive HIV test result?

CITATION:
Govender RD, Schlebusch L, Esterhuizen T. Brief suicide preventive intervention in newly diagnosed HIV-positive persons. Submitted to the *African Journal of Psychiatry* for consideration.

ABSTRACT:
Background. In South Africa, suicide rates range from 11.5 to 25/100 000 among the general population with non-fatal suicides occurring predominantly among females. South African studies have found that people diagnosed with HIV/AIDS have an increased suicide risk.
Objective. We evaluated the effect of a brief psychosocial intervention on

suicide risk following a positive HIV-test result.

Methods. The study was conducted at a university-affiliated hospital in Durban, KwaZulu-Natal, South Africa. Consenting adult patients (age 18 years and older) diagnosed as being HIV-positive following VCT were enrolled in the study. Participants (N=126) were assigned to SPTC; thereafter, every alternate patient was counselled using a BSPI. Patients were assessed at baseline, 72 hours and 6 weeks after a positive HIV-test result.

Results. Sixty-two participants received SPTC only (control group), whereas 64 were also subjected to the BSPI (intervention group). The crude incidence rate ratio for suicidal ideation for the BSPI, compared with SPTC only, was 0.80 (95% CI 0.52 - 1.23); therefore, the intervention proved protective against suicidal ideation.

Conclusion. Although both groups benefitted from post-test counselling, results from the BSPI group demonstrated a clinically significant decrease in suicidal ideation over the time period studied. The results provide preliminary evidence on the efficacy of a BSPI for recently diagnosed vulnerable HIV-positive persons and the importance of educating such patients on suicide-prevention strategies.

CHAPTER 5

CONCLUSION

In this chapter, the most significant research findings of the overarching study are summated. The limitations of the research are discussed and recommendations are made for future studies.

5.1 SUMMARY OF THE EMPIRICAL FINDINGS

The overarching aim of this study was to measure the effectiveness of an SRSS among HIV-positive persons, in order to assess and implement a BSPI post VCT to reduce suicidal ideation in recently diagnosed HIV-positive persons.

5.1.1 SUICIAL IDEATION

Of the 157 participants (83.1%) who tested HIV-positive, the risk of suicidal ideation was 20.5% at 72 hours; while 6 weeks thereafter, the risk was 28.8%. Although the number of suicidal patients was the same at both time-points (n=32), only 8 participants were classified as suicidal at both points. There were 23 new cases of suicidal ideation between 72 hours and 6 weeks, i.e. these participants were not suicidal at 72 hours, but became suicidal by the 6-week time-point. This represents a suicidal incidence risk of 20.9% (95% CI 13.97 - 29.92). The incidence of suicidal ideation between 72 hours and 6 weeks was significantly associated with HIV status (p=0.013). None of the HIV-negative patients displayed suicidal ideation after being informed of their seronegative status. Suicidal ideation increased from 17.1% (95% CI 12.16 - 23.45) at 72 hours to 24.1% (95% CI 17.26 - 32.39) 6 weeks thereafter, confirming a significant association between HIV-positive VCT test results and suicidal ideation.

5.1.2 SOCIODEMOGRAPHIC FACTORS

The mean age was 33.49 years (SD ±9.449) for HIV-positive patients and 37.94 years (SD ±15.238) for HIV-negative patients, with a participant age range of 16 - 79 years. The majority of participants (38.5%) fell within the 21 - 30-year age category. Despite the fact that a wide age range was represented in the cohort, the majority of seropositive patients with suicidal ideation fell within the younger age group (age <30 years), consistent with the age-related spread of the disease and the increase in suicidal behaviour in younger people. The sample comprised 70.8% females and 59.4% unemployed individuals.

HIV-positive respondents showed a significantly increased risk of suicidal ideation at both time-points (72 hours and 6 weeks), associated with increasing age. As age increased by one year, the risk of being suicidal increased by a factor of 1.03 (95% CI 1.005 - 1.059; p=0.020 and p<0.001, respectively). At 6 weeks, both age and gender were significant predictors of suicidal ideation with males having a 1.8 times higher risk of suicidal ideation than females (p=0.025). No other demographic variable was significantly associated with suicidal ideation at 6 weeks.

Table 1. Suicidal ideation according to age and gender

	Age; 72 h	Age; 6 weeks	Gender; 6 weeks	
Risk ratio	1.031831	1.03143	1.783475	
Standard error	0.0139276	0.00722	0.4616398	
z	2.32	4.42	2.24	
$p>|z|$	0.020	0.000	0.025	
95% CI	1.004892	- 1.017376	- 1.07384	-
	1.059493	1.045678	2.962064	

Age was the only significant risk factor for incidence of suicidal ideation between 72 hours and 6 weeks (RR 1.05; 95 % CI 1.037 - 1.063; p<0.001).

The risk for HIV seropositivity correlated with a greater number of females testing HIV-positive. Age was a significant factor in that for each year increase in age, the risk of testing HIV-positive decreased by 4.1%. A lower level of education and the presence of traditional beliefs were also significantly associated with testing HIV-positive.

5.1.3 HOPELESSNESS AND DEPRESSION

Thirty-two HIV-positive participants (20.5%) had a hopelessness score of greater than or equal to 9 on BHS at 72 hours after HIV diagnosis, and 32 (28.8%) had a score in this range at 6 weeks. These findings demonstrate an increase in hopelessness over 6 weeks; and importantly, many studies have shown that hopelessness correlates with the risk for suicide. One hundred and thirty HIV-positive participants (82.8%) were depressed according to the BDI scores at 72 hours after diagnosis, while 86 (78.2%) were depressed at 6 weeks. The average BDI scores were 15.20 and 14.23, respectively, at the two time-points. Pearson's correlation coefficients for the hopelessness and depression scores were 0.556 (p<0.001) at 72 hours and 0.625 (p<0.001) 6 weeks after diagnosis, illustrating a moderately positive correlation at both points.

Although research in high income countries has shown that suicidal patients are depressed (Cooper-Patrick L, *et al.*, 1994; Wolfersdorf M, 2008), the results in this study has shown an opposing trend where depression decreased over the 6 week period while suicidal ideation increased over the same period.

'My future looks dark' is the statement representing item 7 of BHS. The mean scores for this item were 0.561 at 72 hours and 0.421 at 6 weeks. At 72 hours, 28% of the respondents who endorsed this statement had a score sufficiently high and statistically significant (p=0.002) to predict suicidal ideation. At 6 weeks, 57% of the respondents endorsed this item, confirming a predisposition for suicidal ideation, with a statistically significant association (p<0.001).

Item 9 of BDI is represented by the following options: 'I don't have any thoughts of killing myself', 'I have thoughts of killing myself, but I would not carry it out', 'I would like to kill myself' and 'I would like to kill myself if I had the chance'. The mean scores for this item were 0.154 at 72 hours and 0.076 at 6 weeks. A significant association was shown between the responses to this item and suicidal ideation as defined by BHS (by the standard cut-off scores), with p-values of 0.036 and 0.008 at 72 hours at 6 weeks, respectively; 36% and 66% of the patients showed evidence of suicidal ideation on both item 9 of BDI and on BHS at both time-points.

The AUC of the ROC curve of the BDI scores used to predict suicidal ideation was 0.757 (p<0.001) at 72 hours and 0.788 (p<0.001) at 6 weeks, indicating that the BDI score was a good predictor of suicidal ideation, and proving the strong correlation between hopelessness, depression and suicidal ideation. These results support the evidence of previous studies   (Chiles JA, *et al.*, 1989; Beck AT, *et al.*, 1993; Priester and Clum, 1992).

5.1.4 SUICIDE RISK SCREENING SCALE

A 14-item, self-administered scale (*section 3.3, Chapter Three*), developed from 11 items of BHS and 1 item from BDI, was used to screen for suicidal ideation in recently diagnosed HIV-infected persons. The cut-off score of 4 and above demonstrated 68% sensitivity and 64% specificity in predicting suicidal ideation. Ideally, the test should be more sensitive than specific to identify as many probable suicidal patients as possible, hence the basis of our rationale for maximising sensitivity in this analysis. The AUC in ROC analysis was 0.730 at baseline (95% CI 0.64 - 0.81) and 0.776 at 3 weeks (95% CI 0.68 - 0.87).

The validity of the SRSS was determined by comparing it with the accepted instrument for SUPRE-MISS. Using a cut-off score of 4, the sensitivity of the SRSS at baseline was 81% with a positive predictive value of 48%, a specificity of 47% and a negative predictive value of 80%. At 3 weeks, the sensitivity was 79%, the specificity 55%, the positive predictive value 44%, and the negative predictive value 82%. The overall Cronbach's alpha for the SRSS at baseline and at 3 weeks was 0.874 and 0.915, respectively, suggesting that the SRSS is a valuable screening tool for detecting suicidal ideation among patients attending VCT clinics.

5.1.5 BRIEF SUICIDE PREVENTIVE INTERVENTION

Twenty-four (38.7%) participants in the SPTC group were determined to have features of hopelessness at baseline; this was reduced to 5 (8.1%) participants after 72 hours, and increased to 11 (18.3%) after 6 weeks. The BSPI group showed a similar trend with 21 (32.8%) initially, 5 (7.8%) 72 hours later and 8 (12.7%) after 6 weeks. The direct suicide risk in both the SPTC and BSPI groups, respectively, was 11.5% and 10.9% at baseline, and 3.2% and 1.6% at 72 hours; none were suicidal at 6 weeks. Upon assessment of suicidal ideation among participants following SPTC (*n*=37) and BSPI (*n*=32) at the three time-points (baseline, 72 hours and 6 weeks after a positive HIV-test result), the intervention group showed a lower prevalence of suicidal ideation than the control group.

The crude incidence rate ratio for suicidal ideation for the intervention group was 0.80 (95% CI 0.52 - 1.23). Upon comparison of this ratio with that of the control group, the intervention was deemed protective against the incidence of suicidal ideation. There was a highly significant change from being positive (suicidal ideation) to negative (no suicidal ideation) from baseline to 72 hours thereafter. The BSPI was shown to be highly effective in reducing suicidal ideation, especially in the first 72 hours following a positive HIV diagnosis.

5.2 STUDY CONTRIBUTIONS

This study is the first of its kind conducted in South Africa. It has been invaluable in establishing baseline data on suicidal ideation in recently diagnosed HIV-positive persons in KwaZulu-Natal Province. No research previously focused on assessing suicidal risk in HIV-positive persons with the objective of implementing an appropriate suicide preventive intervention.

This research saw the development of a self-administered, quick and simple screening scale to identify HIV-positive patients at high risk for suicidal ideation. The newly developed and tested SRSS may be used in under-resourced settings without the need for additional trained staff. It is easily scored (with TRUE=1 and FALSE=0), with an overall score of 4 and above indicative of a high risk for suicidal ideation. Many similar studies have shown the effectiveness of brief interventions for alcohol and drug abuse (Kypri *et al.*, 2008; Winters *et al.*, 2012).

The rationale of this research was to implement a BSPI immediately following a positive HIV diagnosis, as this would be the most opportune time to administer such an intervention. The implementation of a BSPI with the SPTC was shown to decrease suicidal ideation, particularly within the first 72 hours after conveyance of a positive HIV diagnosis. We can consider these first 72 hours as the 'golden hours of suicide prevention' in HIV-positive persons; all patients who are lost to follow-up would still have the benefit of suicide intervention. Particularly within the South African context, this is an absolute advantage.

In the resource-limited context of South Africa, suicide risk assessment and interventions are limited by a shortage of adequately trained healthcare professionals, suicide risk screening in general, and guidelines for suicide preventive interventions. HIV counsellors are typically responsible for pre- and post-test HIV counselling and psychosocial education, and they can easily be task-shifted to screen for suicide risk and provide suicide interventions. At a reasonable cost and with minimal training, this approach would see the effective reduction of suicidal ideation.

5.3 STUDY LIMITATIONS

Several limitations of this research warrant discussion. The overall study's generalisability needs to be considered. The sample sizes were not large and the overall study was confined to the post-HIV-test period, with the target part of the population being urban-based. Thus, the results should be interpreted with caution. Other variables which were not measured in the study could have affected the outcomes, e.g. there was no information on pre-existing psychiatric disorders, previous suicide attempts or family history of suicide, and this restricted more in-depth exploratory analyses. Furthermore, in some instances it may be considered more insightful to explore participants who have had related experiences with suicide, e.g. participants who have previously attempted suicide or who have previously had suicidal ideation. Although this may provide valuable insight into suicidal behaviour in general, generalisations would be more difficult to make if such participants formed the bulk of the study cohort.

It must be noted that suicide data is obtained from a research-based database, the South African National Injury Mortality Surveillance System (NIMSS) (NIMSS, 2007), and data from the Durban Parasuicide Study (PDS) (Schlebusch, 2004). These data bases are not accurate for many reasons and the NIMSS is bias towards the urban areas. South Africa post-1994, is presently updating its previously 4 data bases to compiling a single, comprehensive one. Therefore the national statistics are a rough estimate and should be interpreted with caution.

Although Beck's cognitive model has been has been confirmed by multiple studies, it has to be used with caution because the relationship among suicidal behaviour, depression, and hopelessness has been shown to be affected by the cultural, demographic, and psychological factors.

Weaknesses in the study design must be noted. In this context, the relationship between seropositivity, hopelessness, depression and ultimate suicide could not be assessed for ethical reasons. An added limitation and due to ethical constraints, is that pre-test assessments were not done which would have strengthened the hypothesis testing.

The construction of the SRSS involved selecting items from two sub-scales, which were grouped and analysed as a single scale. Although the SRSS has potential to be utilised as a simple screening tool to detect suicidality in HIV-infected individuals, it needs to be further evaluated in future research. Moreover, challenges arose with the lack of a gold standard against which the SRSS could be validated. The SRSS assesses hopelessness as a mediator for suicidal ideation and therefore indirectly evaluates participants' views about their positive HIV diagnosis, although it would have been more useful to assess the participants' views on living with HIV directly. This information could form part of a clinical interview in future research.

Importantly, time is a consideration in determining outcome. In the intervention study, the follow-up period was only 6 weeks; consequently, it is uncertain as to whether the BSPI could sustain significant long-term outcomes. More rigorous, longitudinal and controlled studies need to be conducted to delve into this aspect of the intervention.

5.4 RECOMMENDATIONS AND FUTURE RESEARCH

This research is novel exploring the relationship between hopelessness, depression and suicidal ideation using a theoretical model based on Beck's cognitive model within a multicultural, HIV-infected cohort. It is recommended that further research into the structural relationships between depression, hopelessness, and suicidal ideation be evaluated as originally suggested.

The results from this research support the use of a SRSS and BSPI in HIV-positive persons following a positive HIV diagnosis. It is recommended that this should become routine comprehensive care.

Researchers agree that suicidal behaviour is a multifaceted and complex phenomenon. It is consequently important that researchers gain greater clarity concerning the length of time that an individual may be deemed to be at risk for suicidal ideation and behaviour following a traumatic event such as being diagnosed HIV-positive. In a review of 36 randomised controlled trials of screening and brief intervention for hazardous drinking, interventions were shown to be effective for 12 months or longer (Kypri K et al., 2008). Longitudinal studies are therefore recommended to determine the effectiveness of screening and BSPIs for HIV-infected persons over various follow-up time periods.

It is further recommended that suicidal ideation should be explored with due consideration for additional variables, including: a family history of suicide; a past history of suicide attempts; specific personality traits; and the combination of risk and protective factors as determinants of suicidal ideation. Longitudinal studies are

~ 51 ~

recommended to enable researchers to observe and differentiate between the variables that are more prevalent at different stages of the disease, as well as the impact of the introduction, and even discontinuation of ARVs on suicidal behaviour.

It is recommended that screening for suicide risk should include clinical interviews in addition to a questionnaire-based approach, especially for those patients who are deemed to be at high risk for suicidal behaviour. Comparative research encompassing these two screening approaches may provide invaluable insights into their effect on the intervention outcome.

For future evaluation of the BSPI, a clinical trial is recommended.

Going forward, further research should be embarked upon to explore suicidal behaviour in HIV-positive persons in the context of changing suicidal behaviour patterns and to explore other variables that may influence suicidal behaviour – especially in the milieu of ARV treatment, and considering that 2014 represents 10 years since the public sector rollout of antiretroviral therapy in South Africa.

REFERENCES

Abbey JG, Rosenfeld B, Pessin H, Breitbart W. Hopelessness at the end of life: The utility of the hopelessness scale with terminally ill cancer patients. Br J Health Psychol 2006; 11(2): 173-183.

Abramson LY, Metalsky GI, Alloy LB. Hopelessness depression: A theory-based subtype of depression. Psychological Review 1989; 96(2):358-372.

Abramson LY, Alloy LB, Metalsky GI. The hopelessness theory of depression: Current status and future directions. In: Stein NL, Leventhal, B, Trabasso T, eds. Psychological and Biological Approaches to Emotion. Hillsdale, NJ: Lawrence Erlbaum Associates, 1990: 333-358.

Acturial Society of South Africa (ASSA). ASSA 2008 AIDS and Demographic Model (lite version 110207).

Pretoria: ASSA, 2011. http://aids.actuarialsociety.org.za/ASSA2008-Model-3480.htm (accessed 16 July 2013).

Aish AM, Wasserman D. Does Beck's Hopelessness Scale really measure several components? Psychol Med 2001; 31: 367-272.

Allen JP. An Overview of Beck's Cognitive Theory of Depression in Contemporary Literature. http://www.personalityresearch.org/papers/allen.html (accessed 26 August 2013).

American Psychiatric Association (APA). Diagnostic and Statistical Manual of Mental Disorders, Fourth Edition, Text Revision (DSM-IV-TR). Arlington, VA, USA: APA, 2000.

American Psychiatric Association (APA). Handbook of Psychiatric Measures. Washington, DC, USA: APA, 2000.

AVERT. Worldwide HIV & AIDS Statistics. http://www.avert.org/worldwide-hiv-aids-statistics.htm (accessed 6 August 2012).

Badiee J, Moore DJ, Atkinson JH, et al. Lifetime suicidal ideation and attempt are common among HIV+ individuals. J Affect Disorders 2012; 136(3): 993-999.

Bantjies J, Van Ommen C. The development and utilisation of a suicide risk assessment interview schedule. S Afr J Psychol 2008; 38(2): 391-411.

Beck AT. The evolution of the cognitive model of depression and its neurobiological correlates. Am J Psychiatry 2008; 165: 969-977.

Beck AT, Brown G, Berchick RJ, et al. Relationship between hopelessness and ultimate suicide: A replication with psychiatric outpatients. Am J Psychiatry 1990; 147(2): 190-195.

Beck AT, Steer RA, Ball R, Ranieri W. Comparison of Beck Depression Inventories -IA and -II in psychiatric outpatients. J Pers Assess 1996; 67(3): 588-597.

Beck AT, Steer RA, Beck JS, Newman CF. Hopelessness, depression, suicidal ideation and clinical diagnosis of depression. Suicide Life Threat Behav 1993; 23(2): 139-145.

Beck AT, Weissman A, Lester D, et al. The measurement of pessimism: The Hopelessness scale. J Consult Clin Psych 1974; 42: 861-865.

Bertolote JM, Fleischmann A, De Leo D, et al. Suicidal attempts, plans and ideation in culturally diverse sites: The WHO SUPRE-MISS community survey. Psychol Med 2005;35:1457-1465.

Bertolote JM, Fleischmann A. A global perspective on the magnitude of suicide mortality. In: Wasserman D, Wasserman C, Eds. Oxford Textbook of Suicidology and Suicide Prevention. A Global Perspective Oxford: Oxford University Press, 2009: p. 91-98.

Blakely TA, Collings SCD, Atkinson J. Unemployment and suicide. Evidence for a causal association? J Epidemiol Community Health 2003;57 594-600.

Brown GW, Harris T. Social origins of depression. New York: Free Press. 1978.

Carrico AW. Elevated suicide rate among HIV-positive persons despite benefits of antiretroviral therapy: Implications for a stress and coping model of suicide. Am J Psychiatry 2010; 167: 117-119.

Carrico AW, Johnson MO, Morin, et al. Correlates of suicidal ideation among HIV-positive persons. AIDS 2007; 21(9): 1199-1203.

Catalan J, Harding R, Sibley E, et al. HIV infection and mental health: Suicidal behaviour – systematic review. Psychol Health Med 2011; 16(5): 588-611.

Chiles JA, Strosahl KD, Ping ZY, et al. Depression, hopelessness and suicidal behavior in Chinese and American psychiatric patients. American Journal of Psychiatry 1989; 146, 339–344.

Ciesla GR, Roberts JE. Meta-analysis of the relationship between HIV infection and risk for depressive disorders. Am J Psychiatry 2001; 158: 725-730.

Cooperman NA, Simoni JM. Suicidal Ideation and Attempted Suicide Among Women Living With HIV/AIDS. Journal of Behavioral Medicine 2005; 28 (2): 149-155.

Cooper-Patrick L, Crum RM, Ford DE. Identifying suicidal ideation in general medical patients. JAMA 1994; 272(22):1757-1762.

De Leo D, Bertolote JM, Kerkhof AJFM, et al. Definitions of Suicidal Behaviour. Lessons learnt from the WHO/EURO Multicentre Study. Crisis 2006; 27(1): 4-15

Dyer JAT, Kreitman N. Hopelessness, depression and suicide intent in parasuicide. British Journal of Psychiatry 1984; (144): 127–133.

Fernandez-Pol B. Characteristics of 77 Puerto Ricans who attempted suicide. American Journal of Psychiatry 1986; 143:1460–63

Fukuchi N, Kakizaki M, Sugawara Y, et al. Association of marital status with the incidence of suicide: A population-based Cohort Study in Japan (Miyagi cohort study). Journal of Affective Disorders 2013; 150 (3): 879-885.

Govender RD, Schlebusch L. Suicidal ideation in seropositive patients seen at a South African HIV voluntary counseling and testing clinic. Afr J Psych 2012; 15: 94-98.

Hankin BL, Abramson LY. Development of gender differences in depression: An elaborated cognitive vulnerability–transactional stress theory. Psychological Bulletin 2001;127(6) : 773-796.

Hatton CL, Valente SM, eds. Suicide Assessment and Intervention. 2nd ed. Englewood Cliffs, NJ, USA: Prentice-Hall, Inc., 1989: p. 43.

Hosegood V, Timaeus IM. HIV/AIDS and Older People in South Africa. In:

National Research Council (US) Committee on Population; Cohen B, Menken J, editors. Aging in Sub-Saharan Africa: Recommendation for Furthering Research. Washington (DC): National Academies Press (US); 2006.

Hoven CW, Wasserman D, Wasseman C, et al. Awareness in nine countries: A public health approach to suicide prevention. Legal Medicine 2009; 11(1): S13-S17.

Joint United Nations Programme on HIV/AIDS (UNAIDS). 2006 Report on the Global AIDS Epidemic, Annex 2: HIV and AIDS Estimates and Data. Geneva, Switzerland: UNAIDS, 2006.

Joint United Nations Programme on HIV/AIDS (UNAIDS). HIV/AIDS Estimates 2012: South Africa. Geneva, Switzerland: UNAIDS, 2012. http://www.unaids.org/en/regionscountries/countries/southafrica/ (accessed 6 August 2012).

Kapci EG, Cramer D. The mediation component of the hopelessness depression in relation to negative life events. Counselling Psychology Quarterly 2000; 13 (4): 413-423.

Kelly B, Raphael B, Judd F, et al. Suicidal Ideation, Suicide Attempts, and HIV Infection. Psychomatics 1998; 39: 405-415.

Kinyanda E, Hoskins S, Nakku J, et al. The prevalence and characteristics of suicidality in HIV/AIDS as seen in an African population in Entebbe district, Uganda. BMC Psychiatry 2012; 12: 63.

Kypri K, Langley JD, Saunders JB, et al. Randomized controlled trial of web-based alcohol screening and brief intervention in primary care. Arch Intern Med 2008; 168(5): 530-536.

Leclerc-Madlala S. Youth, HIV/AIDS and the importance of sexual culture and context. Social Dynamics 2002; 28(1): 20-41.

Lloyd C. Life events and depressive disorder reviewed: I. Events as predisposing factors. Archives of General Psychiatry 1980a 37: 529-535.

Lloyd C. Life events and depressive disorder reviewed: H. Events as precipitating factors. Archives of General Psychiatry 1980b; 37: 541-548.

Mann J, Apter A, Bertolote J, et al. Suicide Prevention Strategies: A Systematic

Review. JAMA. 2005;294(16):2064-2074.

Meel BL, Leenaars AA. Human immunodeficiency virus (HIV) and suicide in a region of Eastern Province ("Transkei"), South Africa. Arch Suicide Res 2005; 9(1): 69-75.

Mhlongo T, Peltzer K. Parasuicide among youth in a general hospital in South Africa. Curationis 1999; 22(2): 72-76.

Morrell R. Gender, Sexuality and HIV/AIDS: Research and Intervention in Africa. Institute of Public Health, University of Copenhagen, Denmark, 23 - 24 April 2001.

National Department of Health (NDoH). National HIV and Syphilis Prevalence Survey South Africa 2006: Summary Report. Pretoria, South Africa: NDoH, 2007.

National Injury Mortality Surveillance System (NIMSS). A profile of fatal injuries in South Africa. 7th Annual Report. Pretoria, South Africa: NIMSS, 2005. http://www.doh.gov.za/docs/report/2007/nimss/sec1a.pdf (accessed 9 July 2013).

Nock MK, Borges G, Bromet EJ, et al. Cross-national prevalence and risk factors for suicidal ideation, plans and attempts. The British Journal of Psychiatry 2008;192: 98-105.

Nordentoft M. Crucial elements in suicide prevention strategies. Prog Neuropsychopharmacol Biol Psychiatry 2011; 35(4): 848-853.

Olley BO, Seedat S, Nei DG, et al. Predictors of major depression in recently diagnosed patients with HIV/AIDS in South Africa. AIDS Patient Car STDs 2004; 18: 481-487.

Priester MJ, Clum GA. Attributional style as a diathesis in predicting depression, hopelessness, and suicide ideation in college students. Journal of Psychopathology and Behavioural Assessment 1992; 14(2): 111-122.

Perry S, Jacobsberg L, Fishman B. Suicidal ideation and HIV testing. JAMA 1990; 263(5): 679-682.

Rehse B, Pukrop R. Effects of psychosocial interventions on quality of life in adult cancer patients: Meta analysis of 37 published controlled outcome studies. Patient Education and Counseling 2003; 50: 179-186.

Rochat TJ, Bland RM, Tomlinson M, Stein A. Suicide ideation, depression and

HIV among pregnant women in rural South Africa. Health 2013;5(3A):650-661.

Robertson K, Parsons TD, Van der Horst C, Hall C. Thoughts of death and suicidal ideation in nonpsychiatric human immunodeficiency virus seropositive individuals. Death Stud 2006; 30(5): 455-469.

Schlebusch L. Current Perspectives on Suicidal Behaviour in South Africa. In: Suffle S, Van Niekerk A, Duncan D, eds. Crime, Violence and Injury Prevention in South Africa: Developments and Challenges. Tygerberg, South Africa: Medical Research Council-UNISA, 2004: p. 88-113.

Schlebusch L. Suicidal Behaviour in South Africa. Andrea Nattrass. Durban: University of KwaZulu-Natal Press, 2005.

Schlebusch L. HIV/AIDS and the risk of suicidal behaviour. Suicidology 2006; 3: 30-32.

Schlebusch L, Govender RD. Age, gender and suicidal ideation following voluntary HIV counseling and testing. Int J Environ Res Public Health 2012; 9: 521-530.

Schlebusch L, Vawda N. HIV-infection as a self-reported risk factor for attempted suicide in South Africa. Afr J Psychiatry 2010; 13(4): 280-283.

Skinner D, Mfecane S. Stigma, discrimination and the implications for people living with HIV/AIDS in SA. J

Soc Aspects of HIV/AIDS 2004; 1(3): 157-164.

Sontag S. AIDS and its Metaphors. London, UK: Penguin Press, 1988.

Treatment Action Campaign (TAC). Mourn Mpho Motloung! Change HIV/AIDS Messages to Show Hope Now! False Message Increases Violence Against Women. Cape Town: TAC, 2002. http://www.tac.org.za (accessed 9 July 2013).

Wetzel RD, Margulies T, Davis R, et al. Hopelessness, depression and suicide intent. Journal of Clinical Psychiatry 1980; 41: 159–160

Winters KC, Fahnhorst T, Botzet A, et al. Brief intervention for drug-abusing adolescents in a school setting: Outcomes and mediating factors. Journal of Substance Abuse Treatment 2012; 42: 279-288.

World Health Organization (WHO). Suicide prevention (SUPRE). Geneva: WHO,

2008.
http://www.who.int/mental_health/prevention/suicide/suicideprevention/en/index.ht
ml (accessed 22 February 2012).

World Health Organization (WHO). Public health action for the prevention of
suicide: a framework 2012.
http://apps.who.int/iris/handle/10665/75166#sthash.M1QZS3xg.dpuf

Wolfersdorf M. Depression and suicide. Bundesgesundheitsblatt
Gesundheitsforshung Gesundheitsschutz 2008;51(4):443-450.

Yip PSF, Cheung YB. Quick assessment of hopelessness: A cross-sectional study.
Health Qual Life Out 2006; 4(13)

ANNEXURE ONE

SOCIODEMOGRAPHIC QUESTIONNAIRE (ENGLISH)

SOCIODEMOGRAPHIC QUESTIONNAIRE		Computer-generated No.:	
Age:			
Sex:		Male	Female
Educational qualifications:		Primary	
		Grade 8	
		Grade 10	
		Grade 12	
(Tick √ the highest qualification, where applicable)		Diploma (teaching/engineering)	
		Degree (BSc/BComm)	
		None	
Occupation:		Unemployed	
		Scholar	
		Unskilled (gardener/painter)	
		Skilled (technical/diploma)	
		Professional (university degree)	
		Pensioner	
		Other	
Marital status:		Married	
		Single	
		Divorced	
		Living together with a partner	
Cultural group:		Zulu	
		Xhosa	
		Hindu	
		Muslim	
		Christian	
		Other	
If other then specify:			

SOCIODEMOGRAPHIC QUESTIONNAIRE (ISIZULU)

UHLA LWEMIBUZO		Computer-generated No.:	
Iminyaka yobudala:			
Ubulili:	Owesilisa	Owesifazane	
Izinga lemfundo: (Bhala uphawu √ kwibanga lemfundo owalizuza)	Primary Grade 8 Grade 10 Grade 12 Diploma (teaching/engineering) Degree (BSc/BComm) None		
Umsebenzi owenzayo:	Unemployed Scholar Unskilled (gardener/painter) Skilled (technical/diploma) Professional (university degree) Pensioner Other		
Ushadile/ awushadile:	Ushadile Awushadile Wehlukanisile Uhlala ndawonye nomlingani		
Uhlanga:	Zulu Xhosa Hindu Muslim Christian Other		
Isizathu sakho sokufuna ukuhlolwa nokwelulekw:			

~ 61 ~

ANNEXURE TWO
BECK'S HOPELESS SCALE (ENGLISH)

HOPELESSNESS SCALE	Computer-generated No.:	
This questionnaire consists of twenty statements (sentences). Please read the statements carefully one by one and answer them. If this statement describes your attitude *for the past week, including now,* write down 'T' in the block provided. If the statement is false for you, write 'F' in the block provided. **You do not have to answer questions to which you do not want to respond.**		
Statement		**T or F**
1. I look forward to the future with hope and enthusiasm		
2. I might as well give up because there's nothing I can do about making things better for myself		
3. When things are going badly, I am helped by knowing that they can't stay that way forever		
4. I can't imagine what my life would be like in ten years		
5. I have enough time to accomplish the things I most want to do		
6. In the future I expect to succeed in what concerns me most		
7. My future seems dark to me		
8. I happen to be lucky and I expect to get more of the good things in life than the average person		
9. I just don't get the breaks, and there's no reason to believe that I will in the future		
10. My past experiences have prepared me well for my future		
11. All I can see ahead of me is unpleasantness rather than pleasantness		
12. I don't expect to get what I really want		
13. When I look ahead to the future, I expect I will be happier than I am now		
14. Things just won't work out the way I want them to		
15. I have great faith in the future		

16.I never get what I want so it's to want anything	
17.It is very unlikely that I would get any real satisfaction in the future	
18.The future seems vague and uncertain to me	
19.I can look forward to more good times than bad times	
20.There's no use in really trying to get something I want because I probably won't get it	

SCORING

One point is scored each time the respondent endorses the item in the following ways:
(maximum total = 20)

1.	T		8.	F		15.	F
2.	T		9.	T		16.	T
3.	F		10.	F		17.	T
4.	T		11.	T		18.	T
5.	F		12.	T		19.	F
6.	F		13.	F		20.	T
7.	T		14.	T			

0 – 3: None or minimal

4 – 8: Mild

9 – 14: Moderate (May not be in immediate danger, but requires frequent regular monitoring. Is the life situation stable?).

15+: Severe (definite suicidal risk)

BECK'S HOPELESS SCALE (ISIZULU)

NGAPHAMBI KOKUHLOLWA I HIV		
ISILINGANISO SOKUPHELELWA ITHEMBA	Computer-generated No.:	

Loluhla lwemibuzo lunemisho engu 20. Funda umusho ngamunye ngokucophelela, uwuzwisise. Uma umusho uchaza indlela obuzizwa ngayo kuleliviki kuhlanganisa namanje bhala u "T" esikweleni esiqondene. Uma umusho ungelona iqiniso kuwe bhala u "F" esikweleni esiqondene.

Statement	T or F
1. Ngilangazelela ikusasa ngethemba nokuzimisela	
2. Kungcono ngikhohlwe ngoba akukho engingakwenza ukwenza izinto zibengcono	
3. Uma izinto zingahambi kahle, ngisizwa ukwazi ukuthi ngeke zihlale zinjalo	
4. Angazi ukuthi impilo yami yobe injani esikhathini esiyiminyaka elishumi	
5. Nginesikhathi esenele sokwenza izinto engifisa ukuzenza	
6. Ngizimisele ukwenza konke engifisa ukukwenza	
7. Ikusasa alicacile kimina	
8. Nginenhlanhla futhi ngilindele ukuba nazozonke izinto ezinhle empilweni kunanoma yimuphi umuntu	
9. Angiphumeleli futhi alikho ithemba lokuthi ngiyoke ngiphumelele	
10.Izinto esezenzekile zingilungiselele ikusasa	
11.Ngibona ikusasa linokunganami kunokunama	
12.Angilindele ukuthola engikufuna ngempela	
13.Uma ngibuka ikusasa ngilindele ukuthokoza kunamanje	
14.Izinto ngeke zilunge ngendlela engilindele ngayo	
15.Nginethemba elikhulu ngekusasa	
16.Angikaze ngikuthole engikufunayo ngakho angeke ngifune lutho	
17.Ngeke ngikuthole ukweneliseka ngomuso	
18.Ikusasa alisho lutho kimi futhi alinasiqiniseko	

19.Ngilindele izikhathi ezimnandi kunezimbi	
20.Akusizi ukuzama ukuthola engikufunayo ngoba ngeke ngikuthole	

ANNEXURE THREE
BECK'S DEPRESSION INVENTORY (ENGLISH)

Please read each group of statements carefully. Then pick out the one statement in each group that best represents *the way you feel right now.* **This questionnaire will take about 20 minutes to fill. Should you not wish to answer any questions, you have the option not to do so.**

1. I do not feel sad
2. I feel sad
3. I am sad all the time and I can't snap out of it
4. I am so sad or unhappy that I can't stand it

1. I am not particularly discouraged about the future
2. I feel discouraged about the future
3. I feel I have nothing to look forward to
4. I feel that the future is hopeless and that things cannot improve

1. I do not feel like a failure
2. I feel I have failed more than the average
3. As I look back on my life, all I can see is a lot of failures
4. I feel I am a complete failure as a person

1. I get as much satisfaction out of things as I used to
2. I don't enjoy things the way I used to
3. I don't get real satisfaction out of anything anymore
4. I am dissatisfied or bored with everything

1. I do not feel guilty
2. I feel guilty a good part of the time
3. I feel guilty most of the time
4. I feel guilty all the time

1. I don't feel I am being punished

2. I feel I may be punished
3. I expect to be punished
4. I feel I am being punished

1. I don't feel disappointed in myself
2. I am disappointed in myself
3. I am disgusted with myself
4. I hate myself

1. I don't feel I am worse than anyone else
2. I am critical of myself for my weaknesses or mistakes
3. I blame myself all the time for my faults
4. I blame myself for everything bad that happens

1. I don't have any thoughts of killing myself
2. I have thoughts of killing myself, but I would not carry it out
3. I would like to kill myself
4. I would like to kill myself if I had the chance

1. I don't cry any more than usual
2. I cry more than I used to
3. I cry all the time now
4. I used to be able to cry, but now I can't cry even though I want to

1. I am no more irritated now than I ever am
2. I get annoyed and irritated more easily than I used to
3. I feel irritated all the time now
4. I don't get irritated at all by the things that used to irritate me

1. I have not lost interest in other people
2. I am less interested in other people than I used to be
3. I have lost most of my interest in other people
4. I have lost all my interest in other people

1. I make decisions as well as I ever did
2. I put off making decisions more than I used to
3. I have greater difficulty in making decisions than before
4. I can't make decisions at all anymore

1. I don't feel I look any worse than I used to
2. I am worried that I am looking old or unattractive
3. I feel that there are permanent changes in my appearance that makes me look unattractive
4. I believe I look ugly

1. I can work as well as before
2. It takes an extra effort to get started at doing something
3. I push myself very hard to do anything
4. I can't do any work at all

1. I can sleep as well as usual
2. I don't sleep as well as I used to
3. I wake up 1-2 hours earlier than usual and find it hard to get back to sleep
4. I wake up several hours earlier than I used to and cannot get back to sleep

1. I don't get more tired than usual
2. I get more tired than I used to
3. I get tired from doing almost anything
4. I am too tired to do anything

1. My appetite is no worse than usual
2. My appetite is not as good as it used to be
3. My appetite is much worse now
4. I have no appetite at all anymore

1. I haven't lost weight, if any lately
2. I have lost more than 5 kilograms
3. I have lost more than 10 kilograms
4. I have lost more than 15 kilograms

1. I am purposely trying to lose weight

☐ Yes   ☐ No

1. I am no more worried about my health than usual
2. I am worried about physical problems such as diarrhoea, vomiting, pains
3. I am very worried about physical problems and it's hard to think of much else
4. I am so worried about physical problems, that I cannot think of anything else

1. I have not noticed any recent change in my interest in sex
2. I am less interested in sex than I used to be
3. I am much less interested in sex now
4. I have lost interest in sex completely

SCORING

The individual statements are scored from 0 to 3 and the sum total ranging from 0 to 63.

0 – 9: Not depressed

10 – 15: Mildly depressed

16 – 24: Moderately depressed

25+: Severely depressed

NGEMUVA KOKUHLOLWA I HIV

Funda lamaqoqo emisho alandelayo bese ukhetha umusho osho indlela **ozozwa ngayo njengamanje**

1. Angidangele
2. Ngidangele
3. Ngihlezi ngidangele, akupheli
4. Ngidangele kakhulunoma angijabule angikwazi ukubekezela

1. Angilahlekelwe yithemba ngekusasa
2. Ngilahlekelwe yithemba ngekusasa
3. Ngizwa ngingenanto engingayilangazelela
4. Ngibona ikusasa lingenathemba nobungcono angiboni buzobakhona

1. Angiziboni ngiyisahluleki
2. Ngizibona ngihluleke ngokweqile
3. Uma ngibuyela emuva nempilo yami,ngibona ukwehluleka kodwa
4. Ngizibona ngiyisehluleki

1. Ngithola ukweneliseka njengakuqala
2. Angizenameli izinto njengakuqala
3. Angikutholi ukweneliseka kunoma yini njengakuqala
4. Angenelisekile ngako konke

1. Ngizizwa nginecala
2. Ngizizwa nginecala isikhathi esiningana
3. Ngizizwa nginecala isikhathi esiningi
4. Ngizizwa nginecala ngasosonke isikhathi

1. Angiboni ukuthi ngiyajeziswa
2. Kungenzeka ukuthi ngiyajeziswa
3. Ngilindele ukujeziswa
4. Ngizwa sengathi ngiyajeziswa

1. Angiphoxekile ngami
2. Ngiphoxekile ngami
3. Ngenyanyile ngami
4. Ngiyazizonda

1. Angiboni ngimubi ukwedlula wonke umuntu
2. Ngiyazishaya ngobuthaka bami namaphutha
3. Ngiyazisola ngamaphutha ami
4. Ngiyazisola ngakokonke okubi okwenzekayo

1. Angicabangi ukuzibulala
2. Ngiyacabanga ukuzibulala, kodwa kunzima ukukwenza lokho
3. Ngifisa ukuzibulala
4. Ngingathanda ukuzibulala uma nginethuba

1. Angikhali ngokweqile kokujwayelekile
2. Ngikhala ngokudlulela kunakuqala
3. Sengihlala ngikhala
4. Ngangikwazi ukukhala, kodwa manje angisakwazi nakuba ngifuna

1. Angicasukile manje kunokujwayelekile
2. Ngicasuka kalula kunakuqala
3. Ngihlala ngicasukile manje
4. Angisacasulwa yizinto ezazingicasula kuqala

1. Angisabakhathalele abanye abantu
2. Angisabakhathalele njengakuqala abanye abantu
3. Sengilahlekelwe okuningi ukukhathalela abantu
4. Sengilahlekelwe yiko konke ukukhathalela abanye abantu

1. Ngithatha izinqumo ezingcono kunakuqala
2. Ngihlehlisa ukuthatha izinqumo ngaphezu kwakuqala
3. Ngithola kunzima ikuthatha izinqumo kunakuqala
4. Angisakwazi ukuthatha izinqumo

1. Angizizwa ngibukeka kabi kunakuqala
2. Ngiphatheke kabi ukuthi sengibukeka ngigugile ngingakhangisi
3. Ngicabanga ukuthi kunezinguquko ezingqala ezingenza ngingabukeki
4. Ngikholwa ukuthi ngibukeka ngimubi

1. Ngisengasebenza njengakuqala
2. Sekubanzima ukuqala ukwenza nomayini
3. Ngiyazabalaza ukwenza noma yini

4. Angikwazi ukusebenza nhlobo

1. Ngisalala kahle njengokujwayelekile
2. Angisalali njengokujwayelekile
3. Ngivuka kusasele amahora angu 1-2 kunokujwayelekile kungabe kusalaleka
4. Ngivuka kusasele amahora ambalwa kungabe kusalaleka

1. Angikhathali ngokudlula okujwayelekile
2. Ngikhathala ngokudlula okujwayelekile
3. Ngikhathazwa ukwenza cishe noma yini
4. Ngikhathele angikwazi kwenza lutho

1. Angisakuthandi kakhulu kunakuqala ukudla
2. Angisakuthandi njengakuqala ukudla
3. Angisakuthandi kakhulu ukudla manje
4. Angisakuthandi kwasampela ukudla

1. Asikehli isisindo sami
2. Isisindo sami sehle ngokungaphezulu kuka 5 kg
3. Isisindo sami sehle ngokungaphezu kuka 10 kg
4. Isisindo sami sehle ngokungaphezulu kuka 15 kg

1. Ngizama ukwehlisa isisindo sami

☐ Yes   ☐ No

1. Angisayikhathalele ampilo yami njengakuqala
2. Ngiphatheka kabi uma ngicabanga ngezifo ezinjenge diarrhea,ukubuyisa,izinhlungu
3. Ngiphatheka kabi uma ngicabanga ngezifo kulukhuni ukucabanga okunye
4. Ngiphatheka kabi kakhulu uma ngicabanga ngezifo ngendlela yokuthi angikwazi ukucabanga enye into
1. Angikaluboni ushintsho ekuthandeni kwami ucansi
2. Angisalukhathalele njengakuqala ucansi
3. Angisenandaba kakhulu nocansi
4. Angisaluthandi sampela ucansi

~ 71 ~

Study title: Suicidal ideation in patients with HIV/AIDS following voluntary counselling and testing

Principal investigator: Dr R D Govender

Telephone No: 031-260 4485

GREETING

I am Dr Govender and I am presently doing research to find out if any patients who are HIV-positive have thoughts of suicide. Research is just a process to learn the answer to a question and to determine whether there is a link between suicidal behaviour and HIV positivity.

While awaiting your test you will be asked to complete one questionnaire about yourself. You will be asked to return after 72 hours and again at 6 weeks to complete some questionnaires. Although you will be asked to return after 72 hours and again at 6 weeks, should you be agreeable to be interviewed telephonically, this can easily be arranged. Other than your request for a HIV test, no additional tests will be performed. The initial interview should last about 30 minutes and the subsequent interviews should last about 45 minutes. There will be many other patients who will be interviewed as well.

Voluntary counselling and testing (VCT) will include pre- and post-test counselling. This will be conducted by the VCT Counsellor at the King Edward VIII VCT clinic.

YOUR PARTICIPATION IS VOLUNTARY

Your participation is entirely voluntary. You can refuse to answer any questions that you find too embarrassing or personal. Please note you are free to decline to participate or withdraw at any time from the study without suffering any disadvantage or prejudice to you as a patient or to your treatment.

CONFIDENTIALITY

The information you share with me is confidential and you will be identified in the research by a computer-generated number. No person will be able to link your name with this computer-generated number. Once you understand the study and agree to participate, you will be asked to sign a consent form. You should not agree to take part unless you are completely happy with the study and that you have understood the information given to you. The informed consent form will be locked away in a cupboard that will be accessible to the researcher only. No personal information will be disclosed, unless required by the law or if the Ethics Committee requests this information.

RISKS AND/OR DISCOMFORTS

There are no risks to participating in this study. You may be embarrassed, worried or anxious by some of the questions; please remember that you can refuse to answer any questions that you find too embarrassing or personal.

BENEFITS

This study may not help you directly, but may help others in the future. This study may help doctors and other health professionals to render counselling more able to assist other people living with HIV/AIDS. The results of this study will be published.

COST OF THE STUDY

There is no cost to you to take part in the study. As you will be requested to come within 72 hours and again at 6 weeks, you will be given a fee of R60.00 per visit to cover travelling expenses; or, should you wish to have the interview done telephonically, the telephone expense will be borne by the researcher.

COMPENSATION

You will not receive any financial compensation for taking part in this study.

CONSENT

You are required to sign a consent form if you agree to participate in this study.

LANGUAGE

NB. A translation into the home language of the patient will also be provided where subjects are isiZulu-speaking.

CONTACT DETAILS OF RESEARCHER(S)

For further information/reporting of study-related adverse events:

Dr R D Govender 031-260 4485

PATIENT INFORMATION SHEET (ISIZULU)

Isihloko socwaningo: Ukuziphatha ngokuyela ngasekuzibulaleni kwbahaqwe yigciwane lesandulela ngculazi kanye nengculazi

Umcwaningi omkhulu: Dr R D Govender

Telephone No: 031-260 4485

ISANDULELO

Ngingu Dr Govender kanti njengamanje ngenza ucwaningo ngokuthi bangaki abane HIV/AIDS asebeke bazama ukuzibulala, nokuthiyini eyenza abantu bafune ukuzibulala.ucwaningo luyindlela yokufunda impendulo yombuzo

Ngesikhathi ulindele imiphumela uzocelwa ukuba ugcwalise amaphepha anemibuzo ehlukene amathathu. Uyocelwa ukuba ubuye emva kwamahora angu-72, nasemva kwamaviki ayisithupha ukuze ugcwalise amaphepha anemibuzo. Nakuba uyocelwa ukuba ubuye emva kwamahora angu-72 nasemva kwamaviki ayisithupha, uma uvumelana nokubuzwa imibuzo ocingweni, lokho kungahlelwa kalula. Ngaphandle kwesicelo sakho sokuhlolwa igciwane le-HIV, akukho okunye ukuhlolwa okuyokwenziwa. Ukuphenywa ngemibuzo kokuqala kuyothatha imizuzu angu-30, bese kuthi okulandelayokuthathe imizuzu engango-45. Baningi nabanye abayophenywa ngemibuzo.

UKUBAMBA KWAKHO IQHAZAAKUPHOQELEKILE:

Ukubamba kwakho iqhaza akuphoqelekile. Ungenqaba ukuphendula imibuzo oyithola inganambithisiseki kuwe. Qaphela ukuthi ukhululekile ukwenqaqba ukubamba iqhaza noma ukuphuma kululuphenyo noma nini, ngaphandle kokulahlekelwa yilungelo lakho lokuthola imishanguzo.

UKUBAYIMFIHLO

Ulwazi onginika lona luyimfihlo kanti uyokwaziwa ocwaningweni kuphela ngenombolo eyokhishwa yi-computer. Akekho oyokwazi ukweyamanisa lenombolo negama lakho. Uma sewazi ngocwanongo, futhi uvuma ukubamba iqhaza, uyocelwa ukuba usayine ifomu elisho ukuthi uyavuma. Ungavumi ukubamba iqhaza ngaphandle kokuba uluthokozela lolucwaningo nolwazi olunikiwe uluzwisisa kahle. Ifomu lokuvuma liyovalelwa endaweni aphephile, kube umcwaningi kuphela oyofinyelela kulo. Ulwazi ngawe ngeke ludalulwe ngaphandle uma loku kufunwa ngumthetho noma yiKomidi Elibhekele ukuziphatha. Uma usitshela ukuthi kungenzeka ukuthi wadlwengulwa, umcwaningi uphoqwa ngumthetho ukuba akwazise ukuthi lokho ngeke kube yimfihlo, ukuze kungaphindi kwenzeke lokho, noma uma kushushiswa lowo owenze lesosenzo. Umcwaningi uphoqwa ngumthetho nendlela yokuziphatha ukuba abike ukudlwengulwa kwabomthetho, nawe akweluleke ukuba wenze njalo.

UBUNGOZI KANYE/NOMA UKUNGAPHATHI KAHLE

Abukho ubungozi akubeni kulolucwaningo. Eminye yemibuzo ingenza ube namahloni noma uphatheke kabi kodwa ukhumbule ukuthi ungenqaba ukuphendula imibuzo ekuphatha kabi.

OKUZUZAYO

Lolucwaningo kungenzeka lungakusizi wean ngqo, kodwa lungabasiza abanye ngomuso. Lolucwaningo lungabasiza odokotela nabanye ongoti amkhakheni wezeMpilo ukuba benze ukweluleka kube ngcono kusizakale abahaqwe yigciwane le HIV/AIDS. Imiphumela yocwaningo iyoshicilelwa.

UKUBIZA KOCWANINGO

Ukubamba iqhaza kulolucwaningo kumahhala. Njengoba uyocelwa ukuba ubuye esikhathini esingamahora angu-72 kanye nasesikhathini esingamaviki ayisithupha, uyokhokhelwa imali engu-R60.00 yohambo, noma uma ufisa ukuphenywa ngemibuzo ngocingo, izindleko zocingoziyobhekana nomcwaningi.

UMVUZO

Ayikho imali oyokhokhelwa yona ngokubamba iqhaza kulolucwaningo.

Kulindeleke ukuba usayine ifomu lokuvuma , uma uvuma ukubamba iqhaza kulolucwaningo.

ANNEXURE FIVE

CONSENT DOCUMENT (ENGLISH)

Study title: Suicidal ideation in HIV-positive patients following voluntary counselling and testing

Consent to Participate in Research

You have been asked to participate in a research study.

You have been informed about the study by **DR R D GOVENDER**

You have been informed about any available compensation or medical treatment if injury occurs as a result of study-related procedures.

You may contact **D R R D GOVENDER** at **031-260 4485** during office hours if you have questions about the research or if you are injured as a result of the research.

You may contact the **Biomedical Research Office** at the Westville Campus on **031-260 4769 or 031-260 4553** if you have questions about your rights as a research subject.

Your participation in this research is voluntary, and you will not be penalised or lose benefits if you refuse to participate or decide to stop.

If you agree to participate, you will be given a signed copy of this document and the participant information sheet, which is a written summary of the research.

The research study, including the above information, has been described to me orally. I understand what my involvement in the study means and I voluntarily agree to participate.

Signature of participant	**Date**

Signature of witness (**Where applicable**)	**Date**

Signature of translator (**Where applicable**)	**Date**

NB: A translation into the home language of the patient will also be provided for isiZulu-speaking subjects.

~ 77 ~

CONSENT DOCUMENT (ISIZULU)

IFOMU LOKUVUMA

Isihloko socwaningo: Ukuziphatha ngokuyela ngasekuzibulaleni kwabane HIV/AIDS

Ukuvuma ukubamba iqhaza ocwaningweni

Uceliwe ukba ubambe iqhaza ocwaningweni.

Wazisiwe ngocwanongo ngu **DR R D GOVENDER**.

Wazisiwe ngesinxephezelo esingakhona noma ukwelashwa uma kungakhona ukulimala okwenzeka ngenxa yenqubo ehambisana nocwaningo.

Ungaxhumana no **DR R D GOVENDER** kulenombolo **031-260 4485** (ngamahora okusebenza) uma unemibuzo noma uma ulimele ngenxa yocwaningo.

Ungaxhumana **neMedical Research Office** eNelson R Mandela School of Medicine kulenombolo **031-260 4769 / 031-260 4553** uma unemibuzo ngamalungelo akho njengomuntu osocwaningweni.

Ukubamba iqhaza kwakho kulolucwaningo akuphoqelekile futhi ngeke ujeziswe noma ulahlekelwe uma wenqaba ukubamba iqhaza noma uyeka sewuqalile.

Uma uvuma ukubamba iqhaza uyonikezwa iphepha elifana naleli elisayiniwe nephepha elinika ulwazi kobambe iqhaza, eliwucwaningo ngokufinqgiwe.

Ngichazelwe ngocwaningo kubandakanya nolwazi olungenhla. Ngiyazi ukuthi ukubamba kwami iqhaza ocwaningweni kusho ukuthi ngizivumela ngokwami ukubamba iqhaza.

Isignesha yobamba iqhaza	**Date**

Isignesha kafakazi **(Uma ekhona)**	**Date**

Isignesha yimhumushi **(Uma ekhona)**	**Date**

~ 78 ~

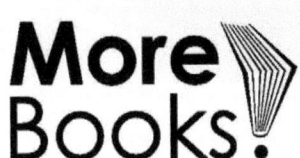
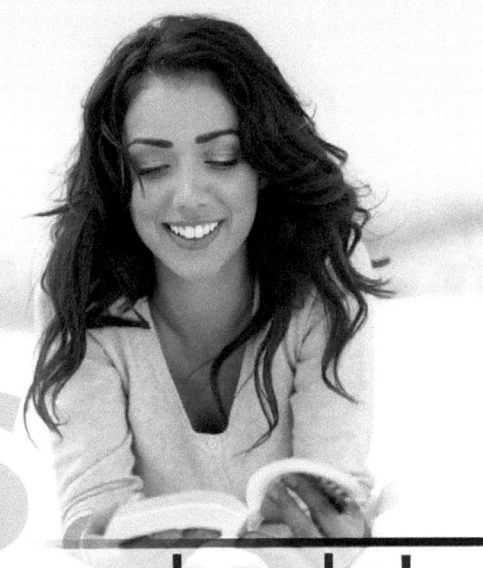 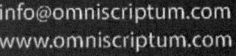
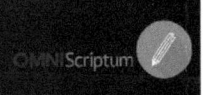

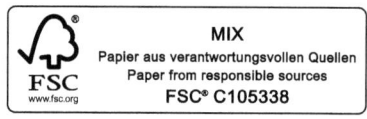
Printed by Books on Demand GmbH, Norderstedt / Germany